OTHER BOOKS BY THE AUTHOR

How to Eat Away Arthritis and Gout
Eighteen Natural Ways to Beat the Common Cold
Eighteen Natural Ways to Beat a Headache
Eighteen Natural Ways to Lower Cholesterol in Thirty Days
Eighteen Natural Ways to Beat Chronic Tiredness
Mind-ing Your Body
Walk to Your Heart's Content
Secrets of Staying Young and Living Longer
Formula for Long Life
Good Health Without Drugs
The Healthiest Places to Live and Retire

D0869310

Acknowledgments

So many sources of pain research were consulted while putting together this book that it is impractical to acknowledge every one. However, I would like to acknowledge the experience and studies of the following institutions and organizations upon which I drew extensively while writing this book:

American Institute of Stress, Yonkers, New York; The Arthritis Foundation, Atlanta, Georgia; Arthritis and Back Pain Center, Santa Monica, California; Center for Exercise Science, University of Florida, Gainesville; Diamond Headache Clinic, Chicago, Illinois; Duke University Arthritis Center, Durham, North Carolina; Hospital for Joint Diseases, Orthopedic Institute, New York City; International Association for the Study of Pain, Boston, Massachusetts; Low Back Pain Clinic, Massachusetts General Hospital, Boston, Massachusetts; Michigan Head Pain and Neurological Clinic, Ann Arbor, Michigan; The Migraine Foundation, Chicago, Illinois; The National Headache Foundation, Chicago, Illinois; National Institute of Arthritis and Musculo-Skeletal Skin Diseases, Bethesda, Maryland; National Institute for Occupational Safety and Health, Bethesda, Maryland; National Institute of Neurological Disorders and Stroke, Bethesda, Maryland; National Institute for the Application of Behavioral Medicine, Bethesda, Maryland; New York Pain Treatment Program, Lenox Hill Hospital, New York City; Northern California Headache Clinic, Mountain View, California; Pain Research Group, University of Wisconsin, Madison; Pain and Stress Therapy Center, San Antonio, Texas; Pain Control Center, Temple University Hospital, Philadelphia; Pain Management Center, University of Texas Health Sciences Center, San Antonio; Pain Treatment Center, Johns Hopkins Hospital, Baltimore, Maryland; Rusk Institute of Rehabilitation Medicine, New York City; Scripps Community Hospital Pain Rehabilitation Center, San Diego, California; The Texas Back Institute, Houston, Texas; University of Miami Comprehensive Pain and Rehabilitation Center, Miami, Florida; Washington University Arthritis Center, St. Louis, Missouri.

I also drew on research or information emanating from such groups as: The Agency for Health Care Policy and Research; American Academy of Neurology; American Academy of Pain Medicine; American Academy of Sports Medicine; American Association for the Study of Headaches; American Academy of Mental Imagery; American Council for Headache Education; American Gastroenterological Association; American Pain Society; American Association of Clinical Hypnosis; and the Association of Academic Physiatrists.

Painstoppers

The Magic of All-Natural Pain Relief

Norman D. Ford

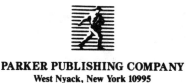

PARKER PUBLISHING COMPANY
West Nyack, New York 10995

10 9 8 7 6 5 4 3 2

Library of Congress Cataloging-in-Publication Data

Ford, Norman D.,
    Painstoppers: The magic of all-natural pain relief / by Norman D. Ford
    p.   cm.
    Includes index.
    ISBN 0-13-143884-0 — ISBN 0-13-143892-1 (pbk.)
    1. Pain—Alternative treatment. 2. Mind and body therapies.
3. Analgesia.   I. Title.
RB127.F663 1994
616'.0472— dc20   93-21418
                                                              CIP

ISBN   0-13-143884-0

ISBN   0-13-143892-1 (pbk.)

Parker Publishing Company
Career & Personal Development
West Nyack, NY 10995

Simon & Schuster, A Paramount Communications Company

Printed in the United States of America

Contents

CHAPTER 12. TAKE THE OFFENSIVE AGAINST PAIN WITH THIS ARSENAL OF PHYSICAL THERAPIES FOR ENDING THE PAIN OF SPECIFIC AILMENTS AND CONDITIONS 209

ABDOMINAL PAINS 210

FIBROSITIS PAIN 213

ANGINA, CLAUDICATION, AND HEARTBURN PAIN 214

Introduction

If you suffer from chronic pain and your doctor has told you that medical science can do no more and you must learn to live with your pain, then this book may bring new hope.

The message of this book is that there very likely *is* something *you* can *do* about your pain. I emphasize the words "you" and "do" because this book is about things you can do to lessen, and even to eliminate, your chronic pain.

The first thing you learn is that while mainstream medicine can work wonders in many areas of medical treatment, providing permanent relief from chronic pain is not an area in which it excels. In fact, if you've been going from doctor to doctor and trying one drug after another, with perhaps one or more surgical procedures thrown in, and you still have your pain, you may well be shopping for relief in the wrong aisle of the medical supermarket.

The branch of medical science that really specializes in chronic pain relief is behavioral medicine. The goal of behavioral medicine is to change the way you feel by changing the way you act (or behave). So if you're feeling pain, *you* may well be able to change that feeling to one of comfort by *doing* something with your mind or muscles. In behavioral medicine, the things *you* can *do* are called *action-steps,* and in this book, action-steps that relieve pain are known as *painstoppers.*

Nowadays, behavioral medicine is practiced by many of the nation's top-ranking pain specialists. And behavioral medicine is *the* most successful pain relief system used in the nation's leading pain and headache clinics. In reality, of course, only you yourself can practice behavioral medicine. So it's up to *you* to *do* what it takes to succeed in overcoming your pain. In most cases, no one else can do it for you.

Enroll at a pain clinic and the doctors' main job is to teach you new ways of behaving that experience has shown to help to relieve your particular type of chronic pain. In other words, pain specialists teach you action-steps that *you* can *do* for yourself to relieve your discomfort.

By describing how to do almost every type of action-step, this book places at your disposal just about every natural pain-relieving technique that is currently used and taught at pain and headache clinics. Depending on whether you suffer from the pain of arthritis or headaches, or lower back pain, or knee pain or whatever, there may be as many as 20 or more different things *you* can *do* to help relieve your pain and stop hurting.

Painstopper action-steps fall into three different groups or classes. First are physical action-steps, each of which is effective for every kind of pain. They are described in Chapter 4. Second are mental action-steps, each of which is also effective for every kind of pain. They are described in Chapters 5, 6, 7, 8, and 13. Third are physical action-steps for the relief of specific pain. Each of these techniques works only for one type of pain, and all are described in Chapters 9, 10, 11, and 12.

To get the most out of this book, I strongly urge you to read Chapters 1, 2, and 3 before trying to relieve your pain with any of the more than 100 painstopper techniques. For best results, you need to use a holistic or whole-person approach. For instance, you should—if possible—use three different painstopper techniques: a physical action-step from the first group, a mental action-step from the second group, and a pain-specific action-step from the third group. For even better results, you can use more than one action-step from each group.

You may not always be able to use action-steps from all three groups. But in most cases you can. And if you do, you will create a comprehensive approach that goes to work on the physical and psychological levels simultaneously. This is true holistic healing in action. And as the book explains, when *you do* things to help yourself, you release invisible sources of inner healing power that double or triple the overall benefit.

This book places powerful pain-relieving tools in your hands. But once your pain is alleviated, I invite you to learn how to *stay* pain-free for the rest of your life. *You* can *do* something about that too. You'll find the answers you need at the end of Chapter 14.

Norman D. Ford
Kerrville, Texas

Chapter 1

Ten Vital Secrets for Overcoming Pain

Has your doctor told you that medical science can do no more and you must learn to live with your chronic pain?

You've seen internists, orthopedists, neurologists, psychiatrists, and even an otolaryngologist. You've taken countless lab tests and injections, tried every pain-killing drug from muscle relaxants to antidepressants and narcotics, and probably had one or more surgical procedures.

Your pain has been medically diagnosed as chronic benign pain syndrome, meaning that it is not caused by any disease, disorder, or dysfunction that is medically treatable.

You have already received any medical treatment your doctor recommended. And he or she has given you medical clearance.

But you still have your chronic pain. If anything, it may be getting worse.

So what went wrong?

The plain fact is that you probably committed one or more of the ten most common blunders made by almost every victim of chronic benign pain syndrome. Many of us, in fact, commit all ten mistakes. And we keep on committing them, often for years.

To save you from making these same blunders, I'm going to give you ten vital secrets for successfully overcoming long-term pain. Some of what I'm about to say may run counter to everything you know, or think you know, about chronic pain. Yet awareness of these facts can save you from draining away any more energy, savings, and resources vainly pursuing relief on the pain merry-go-round.

SECRET #1: Try Shopping in a Different Aisle in the Medical Supermarket

Granted, we all need to have any chronic pain checked out by an allopathic physician (a mainstream medical doctor). And we should undergo any medical treatment or procedure needed to eliminate any danger or impairment to our health.

Yet few of us realize that there are two sides to medical science. On one side is mainstream medicine composed of doctors, hospitals, and pharmaceutical manufacturers. Orthodox medicine does an incredible job in treating injuries, emergencies, trauma, and acute disease. If drugs or surgery or other orthodox medical procedures can offer dependable assurance of permanent and lasting pain relief, I strongly urge you to follow your doctor's recommendations.

But when it comes to actually *relieving* pain—particularly chronic benign pain syndrome—orthodox medicine may not have the answer. If, instead of pain relief, all you are getting from traditional medicine is bills, disappointments, and side effects, it may be time to try medicine's other side.

The other side of the medical coin is known as behavioral medicine. It, also, is practiced by general practitioners, orthopedists, neurologists, physical therapists, and other health professionals, and it is the primary form of medicine used to alleviate pain in the nation's several hundred pain and headache clinics.

But instead of using drugs and surgery, behavioral medicine relieves pain by using action therapy.

The core of behavioral medicine is that you can change the way you feel by changing the way you act. If you're feeling pain, you may be able to alleviate that pain by doing something with your mind or muscles.

Although it seems that all the latest high-tech "miracle" treatments have been developed by mainstream medicine, behavioral medicine has made a mockery of many orthodox medical treatments. Researchers at the nation's leading pain clinics have made astonishing progress in developing natural therapies to relieve pain, even when drugs and surgery have completely failed.

Even medical doctors are recognizing the benefits of behavioral medicine. Several once-popular operations for relieving pain in the back, spine, sinus, face, and gallbladder have proved so ineffective that they are almost obsolete today. Instead of surgery or drugs, many allopathic physicians are now recommending action therapy for the permanent relief of lower back pain.

Although behavioral medicine is practiced by health professionals, it can also be learned and used by anyone. The purpose of this book is to teach you how to use it to overcome chronic pain.

We Overestimate the Power of Drugs

Most Americans also severely overestimate the power of pain-killing drugs. Despite an avalanche of new and expensive drugs to hit the market in recent years, low-cost aspirin still remains the basic nonaddictive drug of choice for pain relief.

Most drugs will relieve pain for a few days. After that, their effectiveness steadily diminishes. Scores of well-documented studies have proved that for long-term use, drugs are among the least effective ways to manage pain.

The side effects of many pain-killing drugs are so destructive that the top priority at all pain clinics is to get the patient off all drugs as soon as possible. One reason is that millions of Americans have become so dependent on, or addicted to, these drugs that continued use has created problems far more disabling than the original pain. Continued reliance on drugs for pain relief often worsens the pain, leading the patient to take ever-stronger doses. And the higher the dose, the more intense the pain. Long-term management of pain with drugs has turned millions of Americans into passive, helpless zombies.

Despite all the media hype and TV advertising, the long-term benefits of many drugs approved for sale in the United States remains unproved. For instance, no medical evidence exists to show that tranquilizers are of any benefit in the long-term management of pain. Yet tranquilizers remain the most widely prescribed pain-killing drug.

The Harsh Side Effects of Drugs

One thing *is* certain, however. Whether you're taking simple analgesics, sedatives, muscle relaxants, antidepressants, beta or calcium channel blockers, anti-inflammatory drugs, or narcotics, all have a depressingly long list of adverse side effects.

A review of the most common side effects of pain-killing drugs would include drowsiness, dizziness, blurred vision, vivid nightmares, breathing difficulties, hallucinations, rashes and itching, vomiting and stomach upset, nervousness, swelling, and convulsions. Long-term use may lead to anxiety or depression, liver damage, jaundice, suppression of immunity, bone loss, insomnia, forgetfulness, elevated blood pressure, intestinal bleeding or even ulcers, anorexia, kidney failure, stroke, or congestive heart disease.

The consensus of most physicians specializing in pain is that drugs are inappropriate for long-term pain relief and that only natural, nondrug therapies can permanently alleviate chronic pain.

Across the nation, the hazards and low efficiency of drug-focused treatment is promoting a renaissance in alternative ways to overcome pain. It is this widespread disenchantment with orthodox medicine that has led to the recognition of behavioral medicine as the therapy of choice for relieving chronic pain.

SECRET #2: Ascertain that You are Looking to the Right Person for Chronic Pain Relief

Betty J. had never had a back problem. But one day she bent down to tie a shoelace and heard something snap in her back. The pain was so excruciating that she had to lie down. She remained in bed for two days. Finally, her daughter drove her to see an orthopedist.

He couldn't help. Nor could a succession of five doctors, three specialists, a disc operation, and 15 different medications.

"For two years I was on the pain merry-go-round," Betty told me during a telephone interview. "I went from one doctor to another constantly looking for help. But not a single doctor could do anything to relieve my pain."

At last, a friend convinced Betty to see a physiatrist, a physician who uses behavioral medicine to rehabilitate patients suffering from chronic pain.

"In a single sentence that physiatrist turned my life around," Betty said. "He asked me what I myself had done to relieve my pain."

Betty was momentarily stunned by the question.

"I realized I had done absolutely nothing to help myself," she said. "I had simply been looking for someone else to relieve my pain."

To overcome chronic benign pain syndrome, the physiatrist explained that we should stop looking for help outside ourselves.

"I learned that the power to relieve pain lay within myself," Betty went on. "Each of us has the power to do more to relieve our pain than any doctor, drug, or operation. When your orthodox medical doctor tells you he can do no more to alleviate your pain, self-treatment is the only answer."

Beat the Agony of Pain with Behavioral Medicine

The physiatrist told Betty that behavioral medicine places enormous pain-relieving power in our hands. As soon as we decide to take responsibility for our chronic pain, and to act to help ourselves, we unlock the ability to tap into the body's five built-in pain-zapping functions.

As the physiatrist explained, these natural pain-relieving mechanisms include the placebo and enabling effects, gaining control over our neurological pain gate, releasing pain-killing endorphins in the brain, and gaining power over pain by learning everything about it. A single one of these pain-zapping functions has been shown to reduce pain more effectively than morphine, while another has the capacity to reduce our experience of any type of pain by approximately one-third.

By enlisting Betty's full and active cooperation, the physiatrist taught her a series of easy exercises and relaxation routines and some mental imagery techniques. While each action-step was designed to alleviate the pain in Betty's back, it also set in motion one or more of the body-mind's built-in pain-zapping powers.

"The overall result was incredible," Betty concluded. "Within six weeks, my pain had completely disappeared. I've never felt better. And the physiatrist says that as long as I practice each action-step regularly, the chance of my back going out again is practically nil."

SECRET #3: Be Willing to Play an Active Role in Your Recovery from Chronic Pain

Pain therapy can be active or passive. A passive therapy is typically based on swallowing a drug or receiving an injection or having something done to you by someone else while you passively do nothing. Passive therapies include taking medications or other substances; undergoing surgery; receiving massage, musculoskeletal adjustments, or acupuncture; or undergoing psychological analysis or counseling.

Certainly these therapies can be lifesaving in many circumstances. But they are frequently ineffective for the relief of chronic benign pain syndrome. In fact, pain researchers have found that delegating responsibility for our chronic pain to a health professional merely creates dependency and initiates a passive attitude that may sabotage genuine natural pain relief.

In glaring contrast, an active therapy forces you to take an active role in your own recovery, and it promotes taking responsibility for your pain and taking back control of your life. Typical action therapies include exercise, relaxation and breathing techniques, biofeedback, applying heat or cold, group therapy, do-it-yourself massage or acupressure, yoga and stretching, upgrading diet and nutrition, using therapeutic mental imagery, repeating affirmations, discarding negative beliefs, and cutting out smoking and other pain-inducing habits.

We are using action therapies like these when we carry out the action-steps described in this book.

Knock Out Pain with a Double Whammy

It's important to realize that each action-step carries a double whammy. First, the action-step itself works to help lessen chronic pain. Second, the very idea of undertaking an action-step releases up to five natural pain-zapping powers within the body-mind.

For instance, weak abdominal muscles commonly contribute to lower back pain. When we strengthen the abdominals through exercise, we are performing an action-step that reduces the likelihood of another attack of lower back pain.

But the very act of doing something to help ourselves also releases several pain-zapping factors built into the body-mind that literally double, triple, or quadruple the painstopping benefits of the exercise alone.

With one possible exception, these incredible hidden benefits cannot be accessed by passive therapies.

But to release these powerful pain-subduing powers, we have to *act*. Behavioral medicine is about acting. To get results, we have to *do* what it takes to succeed at relieving chronic pain. This book can't stretch or exercise or relax or visualize for you. It puts you in the driver's seat, and it's up to you to *act*.

Usually you need to learn only half a dozen action-steps, those that are appropriate to your particular type of pain. Often, you can learn them all in a single evening. With a few days of practice, you can frequently do them all in under half an hour.

Altogether, this book describes 101 of the most successful ways of lessening or stopping pain naturally. All are based on active therapies, and the majority were developed at the nation's top-ranking pain clinics and found to be consistently successful.

While I recommend that anyone with chronic benign pain syndrome consult a pain clinic, often that isn't possible or affordable. Nonetheless, the action-steps taught by the clinics are freely available for anyone to use. This book tells how to use each of these painstopper techniques, without cost and in the privacy of your own home.

SECRET #4: Conquer Pain with Accurate Know-how

All it takes to access the first of your body's built-in pain-relieving powers is to learn how the pain process functions in your body-mind.

Eight months of constant and excruciating neck pain left Penny K. physically and emotionally exhausted. She'd tried everything, from seeing an army of doctors and specialists to taking cortisone injections. When her doctor finally suggested an exploratory operation, she felt totally helpless and depressed.

But a few days later her mood changed dramatically. While waiting in her doctor's office, she picked up a health magazine with a special supplement on chronic pain. One of the articles explained the entire pain process in simple, nontechnical terms.

As she read it, Penny began to feel a growing sense of power. By understanding how her body's pain process worked, she suddenly realized that pain was not the terrifying monster that seemed to dominate her life.

As she grasped the dynamics of pain, she also read of several simple action-steps used by pain clinics to lessen the severity of any kind of pain. It dawned on Penny that she could intervene in her own pain process in ways that no doctor could. The article concluded by saying that each of us has a much greater arsenal of painstopping action-steps available than any physician.

As Penny realized how her own neck pain was being caused, the pain itself began to lessen. Within minutes, she felt more comfortable than she had in months. In fact, she felt so good that she canceled her appointment and drove home.

"The mere act of learning how my pain occurred gave me a tremendous feeling of power and mastery over it," she wrote. "The following day the pain was much less severe. Gradually, day by day, it grew less intense until it finally disappeared altogether."

That was three years ago. And Penny hasn't felt a twinge since.

Defuse Pain by Becoming a Medically Informed Layperson

It's been well known for years that one of the best ways to beat any disease or dysfunction is to become a medically informed layperson, that is, to learn as much as you possibly can about your disorder. The literature is filled with case histories of people who achieved a significant level of control over their pain simply by learning all there is to know about it. One explanation is that, as you read and learn more about chronic pain, it becomes much less mysterious and frightening.

Two recent studies made by Dr. Kate Lorig of Stanford University have scientifically confirmed that acquiring medical know-how creates an enhanced sense of being in power and in control of chronic pain.

The first study—of 501 arthritis patients—revealed that those people who received education about the arthritis process reported a 12 percent decline in pain and an 8 percent decline in depression, while values in the control group, who did not receive instruction, actually worsened.

A second study—of 224 arthritis patients over a four-year period —found that arthritis education was as effective in reducing pain as any of the most common arthritis medications. Moreover, members of the experimental group who received the instruction made 43 percent fewer visits to a doctor during the study period than did members of the control group who received no arthritis education.

Having a basic understanding of the body's pain mechanism is the primary action-step in ridding yourself of chronic pain. This explains why virtually every pain clinic gives each patient a crash course in the anatomy of pain.

So another purpose of this book is to make you a medically informed layperson—at least where pain is concerned. After reading Chapter 2, and the remainder of this book, you may know as much, or even more, about chronic pain than your family practitioner.

Understanding Your Pain Mechanism

You'll find this basic know-how invaluable when using the painstopper action-steps in this book. For example, if you apply heat when you should be applying cold, you could worsen your pain instead of relieving it.

If you're feeling impatient and want to start right in and use an action-step to inhibit your pain, I urge you to resist flipping through these pages. "Page shopping" may be as unrewarding as "doctor shopping."

If your pain is caused by arthritis, for instance, you may wish to skip the chapters on headache, back pain, or other types of pain that don't apply. With these obvious exceptions, I urge you to begin reading this book from the beginning and to read one or more chapters each day until you reach the end.

This is because our most powerful built-in pain reliever is the body's own placebo effect. To tap into this dynamic pain-relieving power requires only that you believe implicitly, and have strong faith, in each action-step you are using.

Since behavioral medicine uses many new and innovative therapies, some of us may regard them with skepticism and disbelief. However, once we have an elementary idea of our own body's pain mechanism, we can immediately see how these seemingly radical action-steps work to diminish pain.

For example, if I said that you could lessen your pain by visualizing a pale-blue square in your mind's eye, you'd probably perceive it as some flaky piece of pop psychology from the 1960s.

But suppose you'd learned in advance that some psychologists have found strong indications that the mind symbolizes pain in a specific shape and color. Although our left brain understands English, the right brain communicates only in symbols. By using symbol language, the right brain can tell the nervous system to inhibit or intensify our experience of pain.

Researchers have found strong evidence that when we visualize a shape and color that is incompatible with the shape and color used by the brain to symbolize pain, the right brain signals the nervous system to inhibit its pain response.

The result: our experience of pain is significantly diminished.

Communicate with Your Pain Mechanism—In Right-Brain Language

Another purpose of this book is to teach you how to "speak" to your pain mechanism using right-brain language. By learning to communicate with your subconscious through symbols, you can direct the nervous system to open or close the "pain gate" through which pain impulses travel to the brain.

For this to be possible, however, requires that we first acquire a basic familiarity with the body's pain mechanism.

Still another compelling reason for familiarizing ourselves with our pain process is to realize that pain is not a physical function. Although a pain may seem to be in the back or neck or shoulder or knee, all pain is actually experienced between our ears. Secret #5 explains why the mind is the most powerful reliever of chronic pain.

SECRET #5: Stop Thinking of Pain as Something Physical

Like most Americans, Harold L. regarded pain as a purely mechanical phenomenon that was always caused by something physical such as a ruptured spinal disc or a brain tumor or terminal cancer.

When an unexplained pain appeared in his left shoulder, and the agonizing pain continued relentlessly for days and weeks, Harold consulted his doctor. Harold felt confident that his doctor would find a mechanical cause for his pain, and would cut it out with a scalpel or blast it away with a powerful chemically active drug.

But after an extensive work-up and lab tests, the doctor could find nothing wrong. And no drug the doctor prescribed seemed to help. So his doctor referred Harold to a pain clinic.

At the clinic, a therapist asked Harold what his pain felt like.

"Like a red-hot dagger plunged into my shoulder," Harold replied.

"What would take the pain away?" the therapist asked.

"A bag of ice cubes cold enough to make my skin turn blue," Harold said.

Harold was instructed to sit down and relax and close his eyes. He was then to visualize, in his mind's eye, a red-hot dagger plunged into his shoulder. Gradually, half an inch at a time, he was to imagine the dagger being slowly withdrawn. When the dagger was completely withdrawn, he was to mentally picture a frigid icebag draped across his painful shoulder. In his imagination, Harold was to "feel" and "see" the ice numb his shoulder until the skin turned blue.

The exercise took only a few minutes. As it ended, Harold realized that, for the first time in weeks, his pain was noticeably less severe.

"Relief won't last forever," the therapist told him, "but whenever the pain returns, you can use this same therapeutic imagery to relieve it."

The Medicine of Tomorrow is Freely Available Today

It took only a single demonstration of the mind's pain-relieving power to convince Harold that pain is a subjective, and not a mechanical or physical, phenomenon.

"Pain is a feeling that hurts," the therapist explained. "It may have seemed as though the pain was in your shoulder. But half of all chronic pain begins in the mind. And every pain is *experienced* in the mind. So, naturally, the mind is key to long-term pain relief."

The ability of the mind to alleviate chronic pain has been demonstrated and documented beyond any question of doubt or debate. When we help ourselves by acting, we access up to five different pain-assuaging powers, all located in the mind. And the same type of mental imagery that Harold used has helped tens of thousands suffering from excruciating chronic pain to become pain-free, often for the first time in years. Psychological therapies like relaxation, biofeedback, and therapeutic imagery are the most widely used, and most successful, therapies employed by pain clinics.

Yet subjective pain relief seems so unorthodox that millions of Americans continue to be skeptical of the mind's ability to relieve chronic pain. Clinging to such outdated beliefs denies a person access to behavioral medicine, the medicine of tomorrow—which is already here and freely available for the relief of pain today.

SECRET #6: Genuine Pain Relief Requires a Whole-Person Approach

Most people don't understand pain—but neither do most physicians. A survey in the *Journal of Clinical Oncology* revealed that only 10 percent of doctors felt that their training in pain control had been good or excellent.

While drugs and surgery come under increasing criticism as modalities for pain relief, researchers at the nation's leading pain clinics have made astonishing progress in developing natural therapies that relieve chronic pain, even when all else fails.

Pain clinics owe their success to using a whole-person approach. Instead of merely treating physical symptoms with operations or drugs, they emphasize the combined role of both mind and body in controlling pain. All large pain clinics provide a comprehensive approach that focuses on a person's fears, feelings, and emotions as much as on torn muscles or damaged cartilage or physical malfunctions.

By combining the skills of doctors from a variety of disciplines, pain clinics provide a comprehensive approach to pain relief that has been tremendously successful.

Enroll at any larger pain clinic and you're likely to be examined by an internist, a physical therapist, an orthopedist, a neurologist, a physiatrist, a psychiatrist, and a nutritionist. By combining their multiple expertise, these specialists are able to provide a solution to chronic pain that considers the body-mind as a single unit. In fact, behavioral medicine is the medical extension of holistic (whole-person) healing.

Exciting discoveries in biomedical research have demonstrated that much physical pain is psychological in origin and that chronic pain is a complex condition that almost always requires a whole-person approach.

For instance, if your back goes out as you lean forward to raise a window at bedtime, it may have more to do with how you felt about your job in midafternoon than with straining a muscle in your back at 11:00 P.M. Like most forms of chronic pain, lower back pain is a whole-person problem.

A disagreement with the boss during the afternoon can trigger your body's fight-or-flight response, a primitive reaction that tenses your muscles for immediate reaction. But unlike our cave-dwelling ancestors, in modern society we can neither fight nor flee. So our muscles remain in a crisis mode, primed with energy that we never use. This keeps the muscles in our back rigid and tense for hours at a time.

The mere act of bending over, or raising a window, is then sufficient to create microscopic tears in our overtensed back muscles. Immediately the muscles go into spasm, placing agonizing pressure on nerve endings. The nerves carry pain impulses to the brain, and we experience the pain in our mind.

Virtually every form of behavioral medicine emphasizes the combined role of body and mind. Consider something as simple as walking. As a physical therapy, a brisk half-hour walk not only tones up the muscles and the cardiovascular system, but the exercise triggers the release of endorphins, one of the body's built-in pain-relieving powers. Endorphins are the brain's own morphinelike pain-alleviating opiates. These molecules bind on to pain receptors in the brain, significantly inhibiting the sensation of pain.

Studies show that brisk walking—a physical action-step—not only reduces the severity of many forms of pain for 12 hours or more, but it also inhibits depression and anxiety, both considered to be in the realm of psychotherapy.

Action-Steps for Mind or Body

This book describes both physical and mental action-steps for relieving pain.

Physical action-steps typically include exercise, muscle strengthening, yoga and stretching, self-massage, heat-and-cold therapy, and nutrition. Many work directly on the pain site and are specific only to one kind of pain. For instance, an action-step to relieve knee pain by strengthening muscles in the thigh cannot be used anywhere else in the body. Using physical action-steps may also call for a certain level of mobility and fitness.

Mental action-steps, such as relaxation training, biofeedback, and therapeutic imagery, can be used to relieve any type of pain from headaches to backache, arthritis, or even terminal cancer. People who are in wheelchairs, or who are injured or paralyzed and unable to move, may still be able to carry out all the mental action-steps in this book. By working on a person's beliefs and emotions to change the course of pain, mental action-steps are at least as successful as physical steps, and often more so.

This book is filled with both physical and mental therapeutic techniques. Some are traditional while others are radically new and unorthodox approaches. Most were developed and tested at university medical centers, or at pain and headache clinics, and the majority form the core of behavioral treatment for chronic pain relief.

SECRET #7: Learn to Unleash Your Mind's Built-in Pain-Zapping Powers

A rapidly growing body of evidence from the leading edge of scientific research is providing intriguing proof of our natural pain-relieving powers.

These powers, four in all, are automatically released whenever we perform any physical or mental action-step. However, to access these awesome powers, we need to learn the keys to turning them on.

Mobilize Your Own Placebo Effect

Numerous studies have shown that pain relief comes not entirely from a drug or operation or action-step but from the belief and faith a person has in it. The placebo effect of almost any action-step boosts its effectiveness by approximately 35 percent, regardless of the actual effectiveness of the therapy. In other words, the placebo effect arises from the faith and belief a person has in therapy rather than from any benefit provided by the therapy itself.

When patients are given a sugar pill and are told it is a powerful pain-relieving drug, approximately 35 percent of the patients will experience a significant decrease in the severity of their pain. Their decrease in pain is approximately equal to the benefit they expected the drug to provide. When strong hope is aroused, the mind works independently of the action-step or therapy to provide additional pain relief from within. Frequently, this inner pain relief is stronger than the pain relief provided by the therapy.

To access this extraordinary power, we need only to have strong hopes and expectations that the action-step, or therapy, we are using will succeed.

Numerous studies show that the placebo effect works best when patients are given a detailed explanation of how their therapy works. Understanding clearly how a therapy intervenes in the pain process creates a powerful and unswerving belief in the patient's mind that the therapy will succeed. In turn, this generates renewed hope and a powerful expectation that we shall overcome our pain.

To release our own placebo effect, we need only to read and understand Chapter 2, which describes the dynamics of pain. Additionally, we need to read how any action-step we are using functions to inhibit or prevent pain.

By mobilizing placebo power, we can increase the effectiveness of medical, or any other kind of treatment by approximately 35 percent. Hospital studies show that patients who clearly understand the effect their therapy has on their ailment recover 30 to 35 percent faster from any kind of pain or disorder, including surgery.

Mobilize Your Enabling Effect

This powerful psychological benefit occurs automatically whenever we learn to attribute success in lessening our pain to our own efforts rather than to any drug or surgery or passive therapy.

The enabling effect works because success breeds success. As soon as we detect a small but noticeable improvement in our pain level, it provides powerful confirmation that:

1. We are able to control our pain.
2. We ourselves can do more to relieve our pain than can any drug or treatment done to us by someone else.

To mobilize our enabling effect, we need only to break down our goal of becoming totally pain-free into a series of small, easy-to-achieve steps.

Suppose that on a scale of 1 to 10 we rate our pain as 10. Instead of reaching for a goal of zero, we set a goal of 9 as our first target. To reach that goal we need to reduce our pain level by only 10 percent. Many action-steps will achieve this target quite quickly.

As we succeed in achieving this small step, the positive feedback that we experience propels us toward the next step, a pain level of 8. Step by step, our enabling effect empowers us to reach a goal of seven—and step by step on down to zero.

Close Your Pain Gate with Counterstimulation

During World War II, pain researcher Henry Beecher found that soldiers wounded in battle needed far less morphine than do civilians with similar wounds. Beecher rightly concluded that the soldiers' minds were filled with anticipation of being sent home on leave, while to the civilians, their wounds were merely an added source of anxiety.

Call it distraction or diversion, but whenever the mind focuses on something more exciting, enjoyable, and important, this counterstimulation overloads the nervous system's "pain gate" and forces it to close. As pain impulses are prevented from reaching the brain, analgesia (freedom from pain) occurs.

Every sports coach has seen a player apparently injured in a game but who was so intent on playing that he or she was able to finish the game. Not until the player reached the locker room did pain occur, and it was discovered that the player had fractured an ankle or wrist.

From these and similar examples, researchers have concluded that our perceptions of pain depend on what our minds are focused on. What would happen to your chronic pain, for instance, if someone phoned to offer you a wonderful, well-paid job provided you could start tomorrow?

As we focus on carrying out virtually any action-step in this book, we divert our attention away from pain to something more challenging and engrossing. As our intense mental activity overloads and closes the pain gate, we may cease to feel or experience pain for many hours to come. Additionally, several action-steps are frankly designed to stimulate sensory overload and to cause the pain gate to close.

Turn on Your Brain's Feel-Good Mechanism

Everyone's heard of "runner's high," an incredible feeling of well-being that begins about 30 minutes into a run. The good news is that you don't have to run to generate this natural high. Thirty-five minutes of brisk rhythmic exercise of any type, from walking to bicycling or swimming, is usually sufficient to generate the same effect.

Here's what happens. After 35 minutes of brisk aerobic exercise, the brain releases clouds of tiny peptide molecules called endorphins. Endorphins are natural morphinelike opiates that switch off pain by binding onto pain receptors in the brain.

Not only do endorphins block pain but they also wipe out depression and anxiety for the rest of the day. They also boost our self-esteem and self-confidence and build a strong self-image.

Understandably, not every pain sufferer is able to use brisk aerobic exercise to switch on the brain's feel-good mechanism. But if not, you can achieve much the same effect by thinking positively or by using action-steps designed to deepen relaxation. Therapeutic imagery can also be used to release our natural morphine supply.

SECRET #8: Don't Mistreat Your Body and It Won't Mistreat You

William J.'s life was an inferno of pain. He felt chronic pain all over his body. From the punishing pain of gout in his big toe to osteoarthritis in his knees to racking pains in his lower back, recurring mixed angina in his chest, and regular bouts of migraine headache, William rarely experienced a pain-free moment.

His only solace was to chain-smoke cigarettes, enjoy half-a-dozen cocktails each day, and overeat on rich and fatty foods. He was 40 pounds overweight, and although only 45, he had to use a walker to shuffle about the house. William took excessive amounts of pain-killing medications, and since he could not work, he was constantly anxious and worried about his finances.

His doctor had already told William that his poor health habits were perpetuating his pain. But William refused to listen. To him, his gout and angina and arthritis had become minor issues. His sole interest lay in relieving the pain without changing his life-style.

In desperation, William went from doctor to doctor to chiropractor and naturopath. They gave him a panoply of drugs and herbs and nutrients. But he refused to listen to their entreaties that he stop smoking and overeating.

Finally, William was referred to a physician who specialized in treating pain.

"You're creating your own personal hell," the physician told William bluntly. "Your excess belly fat places enormous strains on your spine and back muscles. It's a wonder you don't have a pinched nerve or a herniated disc."

In no uncertain terms, the physician told William that his life-style was irreconcilable with pain relief. His excess weight was exacerbating the pain in his back and knees while his excessive smoking was a likely cause of his mixed angina and migraine attacks.

"Virtually all your chronic pain appears to be a by-product of your unhealthful living habits," the physician told William. "I'm almost sure you could become pain-free in three months or so if you would simply stop smoking and drinking alcohol and switch to a healthful diet low in fats and high in fiber. You'd also have to begin a gradually increasing exercise program."

William J. Eliminates Disabling Pain

The doctor's serious tone shocked William into realizing that he *must* stop punishing his body-mind with pain-producing habits.

In a rare burst of motivation, William's mind-set turned from hopelessness to hope. Once at home, he stopped smoking cold turkey. He threw out his alcohol. And he replaced all the rich and fatty foods in his diet with salads and other low-fat dishes.

By the fourth day on his new regime, William felt distinctly better. As his enabling effect continued to boost his motivation, his self-esteem soared and his endorphin output increased. Meanwhile, William read a book that explained the body's pain mechanism.

The book also explained that for millions of years, humans have lived a vigorous and physically active life-style, gathering and raising plant-based foods and eating a predominantly low-fat diet high in fiber. But in just three generations, modern man has degenerated to the life of a couch potato suburbanite. Yet our Stone Age bodies continue to need a vigorously active life-style to stay in shape and to remain pain-free. For our body-mind to function painlessly, we have to use our minds and muscles frequently.

William was so impressed that—with his doctor's permission—he purchased a stationary bicycle and began a gradually increasing exercise program. After four weeks, his gout and angina had both disappeared, and his headaches were also fading away.

As one success propelled him to the next, William became an entirely new person. Within three months, just as his doctor had predicted, his chronic pain had disappeared entirely. Although he still had osteoarthritis, his knees no longer bothered him because the excess weight that overloaded them had disappeared.

"You still need to develop your weak abdominal muscles," the doctor said. "And you must continue your good health habits for the rest of your life."

As the physician told William, when our chronic pain is caused by our own destructive life-style habits, it's invariably more productive to focus on eliminating the *cause* of the pain than it is on trying to relieve the pain.

Forty percent of all Americans are overweight or obese while some 25 percent of adult Americans still smoke. Among chronic pain victims, the proportion is higher. With our doctor's cooperation, most of us can realign our value systems so that we place minimum value on pain-producing habits and maximum value on preserving and maintaining our health.

SECRET #9: Finding Your Way Out of the Pain Jungle

Pain relief doesn't have to cost a fortune. But it can if you're subjected to multiple operations or to one battery of tests after another. Virtually any group of tests will show at least one abnormality. In most cases, it's harmless. But to protect himself against possible litigation, your doctor may order additional tests to check out the abnormality. Almost always, one of these will turn up another abnormality. Usually it, too, is harmless. But that provokes yet more tests.

And so it continues, piling up one astronomical bill after another—while the patient remains trapped in an endless cycle of pain.

One morning, Edward K., a Denver stockbroker, experienced a tight pain in his chest on awakening. The pain was so crushing that he broke out in sweat. It continued for 15 minutes before abating.

Edward lost no time in visiting an internist. An EKG test revealed that Edward had probably had a bout of coronary artery spasm, also known as mixed angina. The internist gave Edward some nitroglycerin tablets to relieve the pain and told him that he might eventually need a bypass operation.

A few days later, Edward noticed his heart was skipping beats. This time, he consulted a cardiologist. Edward was given a heartbeat monitor to wear for 24 hours.

When he examined the monitor's recording, the cardiologist's eyebrows shot up. "We may have to implant a pacemaker," he told Edward. "Meanwhile I'll give you a prescription medication."

Seven days later, after a long walk, Edward noticed large red blotches all over his legs and thighs. Alarmed, he phoned a dermatologist for a consultation.

"You have purpura," the dermatologist said. "The only permanent cure is to operate and remove your pancreas."

Together, the cost for the bypass, pacemaker, and pancreas removal totaled $75,000. Meanwhile, Edward's heart was still skipping beats, and he continued to experience angina and purpura.

Pain Relief Doesn't Have to Cost a Fortune

Back in his cardiologist's office a few days later, Edward was thumbing through a health magazine when he came across an article on mixed angina. The author, a nutritionist, described how a deficiency of magnesium may trigger muscle spasm throughout the body and particularly in the coronary arteries. The writer also stated that skipped heartbeats could also be due to a magnesium deficiency.

Edward mentioned this to his cardiologist.

"Not a chance that your angina is diet related," he was told. "High-tech medicine is the only answer."

On the way home, Edward stopped in at a health food store and purchased a $7 bottle of magnesium aspartate. Immediately, he took a 400-mg capsule and continued taking 400-mg each day.

After about ten days, something curious happened. The purpura blotches faded away. Two days later Edward's heartbeat became regular. And from that time on, his angina also disappeared.

Edward didn't bother to return to any of his three physicians. He kept on taking the magnesium supplements. In three years, not one of his symptoms has returned.

"It seems as if there's a deliberate information blackout about nonmedical ways to overcome pain," Edward said in an interview. "Just seven dollars worth of supplements saved me from angina, an irregular heartbeat, and purpura. But if I'd listened to the doctors, it could have cost me seventy-five thousand."

No wonder pain relief has become a multimillion-dollar industry. Pain is epidemic today. Almost one in five American adults has some form of recurring or persistent pain. Twenty-three million Americans have arthritis. Seventy million suffer from chronic lower back pain, and 13 million are crippled by headaches. Chronic pain disables more Americans than heart disease and cancer combined. Pain is the primary reason why people visit a doctor, and it's the number one reason for taking medication.

It doesn't take charlatans or clinics in Mexico or worthless salves and ointments to relieve us of our hard-earned dollars. There are plenty of legal, scientifically validated medical treatments that do so just as effectively. And none will guarantee to relieve our pain.

SECRET #10: There *is* Hope if You're Willing to Act

I'm not claiming that this book will reverse cancer or arthritis or heart disease or any other disease or disorder. But I do believe that, by using the action-steps in this book, you can beat the agony of most forms of chronic pain. You may not succeed at eliminating the pain altogether. But you can gain control, power, and mastery over your pain. And there's an excellent chance that you can decrease the frequency and intensity of your pain, raise your pain threshold, and reduce your pain to tolerable levels.

I don't claim that it will happen tomorrow or next week or next month. It may take several months of regular daily practice. But every one of us has the potential to tap into our inner resources and to divest ourselves of pain.

At various pain clinics I visited, the slogan seemed to be: "With relatively few exceptions, no victim of chronic pain needs to feel helpless or to be incapacitated."

On several occasions I interviewed people who had arrived in wheelchairs only three to four weeks previously and who were already up and able to walk several blocks at a time.

Naturally, I can't give any guarantees. But each of the action-steps in this book has been tried, tested, and found to be at least 50 percent successful by people who should really know—chronic pain sufferers themselves.

Many action-steps have also been validated by well-planned studies undertaken by prominent scientists with impeccable credentials. Many of these techniques are also in daily use by leading pain clinics. When used with your doctor's permission, they are considered safe and effective.

Be willing to accept the probability that you *can* relieve your chronic pain. Learn and practice the action-steps with enthusiasm, willingness, and dedication. And they should help get your pain under control and aid you in living a normal, satisfactory life.

Chapter 2

CHANGING SELF-DEFEATING BELIEF SYSTEMS

The relentless, grueling pain in his lower back had kept John P. home from work for over a month. His doctor could find nothing organically wrong. Pain-killing drugs had long since ceased to help. Yet it was sheer agony just to move. Each time John considered the possibility of losing his job, his anxiety only intensified the pain.

When his doctor referred him to a nearby pain clinic, John jumped at the chance. As an outpatient, his first step would be to attend a one-day crash course on understanding pain.

At the course, a physician who was a specialist in the treatment of pain explained every detail of the pain process, from the stress that contracted muscles and made them taut to the electrochemical pain messages carried by the nervous system through the neural "pain gate" and into the brain. John also learned how a variety of physical and mental action-steps could be used to intervene at various stages of the pain process to inhibit or block out pain.

At home that evening, John felt as if a great weight had fallen from his back and shoulders. Now that he understood how pain functioned, John realized that he himself possessed the power to exorcise his pain. Chronic pain no longer seemed the mysterious, frightening monster he had once feared. For the first time in a month, John was able to get into bed unaided.

This may sound like science fiction. But next morning John woke up feeling cheerful and refreshed; and the pain in his back had almost completely disappeared. He called the doctor with the good news.

The doctor was not surprised.

"Roughly 1 person in every 20 who attends our pain pathology course is completely cured," he said. "Information and know-how alone are all they need to overcome their fears and change the feelings that were causing their pain."

PAINSTOPPER #1:
Let Knowledge Give You Power over the Pain Monster

The doctor explained that for most pain sufferers, half the battle is won once people understand the modus operandi of their pain mechanism and realize that they have the power to act and overcome their chronic pain.

"The more you know about chronic pain, the less you have to fear from it," the doctor continued. "Most doctors prefer patients who have educated themselves about their pain and disorder. Being informed helps you work as a partner with your doctor, and it helps you evaluate your options and to be involved in decisions."

The doctor also explained that for your placebo effect to function, and help to boost your recovery, it's essential to *believe* in the action-steps you are using. And for that to happen, you must clearly understand how the pain process functions.

This chapter covers much the same ground as the course in pain dynamics taught at most pain clinics. *Thus reading and absorbing this chapter could well be the most important action-step you can take to liberate yourself from chronic pain.*

■ THE GENESIS OF PAIN

Stress occurs when we must adjust to a life event that we perceive as threatening or hostile. Whether we see a particular event as friendly or unfriendly depends on our belief system.

A life event, such as becoming unemployed, is not necessarily stressful. It's how we perceive it that creates stress.

Modern psychology considers that only two basic emotions exist: fear and love. All negative thoughts and emotions arise from perceiving life through a filter of fear-based beliefs. All positive thoughts and emotions arise from perceiving life through a filter of love-based beliefs.

Stress occurs only when we perceive life through a filter of fear-based, negative beliefs. And stress is the underlying cause of some 70 percent of all chronic pain. Virtually all pain in the neck, upper and lower back, and shoulders is stress related and so are most headaches. Such pain-provoking diseases as ulcers, irritable bowel syndrome, rheumatoid arthritis, cancer, and heart disease are also stress related. Overeating in response to emotional stress also leads to obesity, which worsens the pain of osteoarthritis.

From working under pressure to conflicts concerning job, money, or relationships to constantly ringing telephones, traffic jams, waiting in line, and long traumatic drives on the freeway, life today is filled with potentially stressful situations.

Yet they are perceived as stressful only when our belief system is programmed by fear. Here is an example.

Smith and Jones are both employed on the production line at a technically obsolete automobile plant. Inability to compete forces the plant to close its doors permanently, and both Smith and Jones are unemployed.

Through his fear-based belief system, Smith perceives his job loss as a disaster. No other sources of employment exist, and he fears his unemployment will be permanent. He fears that he will lose his home, car, and furniture and that he and his family may have to move in with his parents. As Smith's anxiety over the future deepens, he begins to experience chronic tension headaches and bouts of lower back pain that lasts for days at a time.

Jones, by contrast, perceives his unemployment as a welcome release from a boring occupation and as a heaven-sent opportunity to train for a new career in electronics. Jones never felt better, and he gets up each morning to jog in the park before breakfast.

Self-defeating Beliefs Are the Cause of Stress

Although obviously fictional, this example is repeated in real life thousands of times each day. Both Smith and Jones faced exactly the same situation. But through his fear-based belief system, Smith perceived it as hostile and threatening, while Jones, through his love-based beliefs, perceived unemployment as a welcome, and friendly, opportunity for advancement.

Whenever we perceive a situation as threatening, unfriendly, or hostile, the mind triggers the fight-or-flight response and we experience stress. This is exactly what happened to Smith.

But for as long as we continue to experience positive emotions such as peace, optimism. hope, friendliness, joy, fulfillment, forgiveness, and love, our whole person remains in the relaxation response. We experience a minimum of stress, and the body-mind enjoys optimal wellness and freedom from pain. This is exactly what happened to Jones.

It's unfortunate but true that many people with chronic pain see life as Smith did, and they experience stress, depression, anxiety, and other negative emotions.

Although antidepressants and other psychoactive drugs can provide temporary intervention at this stage, only behavioral medicine has a permanent solution.

Through action-steps such as therapeutic imagery and belief restructuring, behavioral medicine can help us reprogram our belief system so that we perceive life in the same cheerful and optimistic way that Jones did. As we let go of our fear-based beliefs, our stress-related pain often disappears as well.

How Belief Restructuring Relieved Janet M.'s Wrenching Back Pain

Restructuring a belief can be as simple as replacing unforgiveness (a negative, fear-based belief) with forgiveness (a positive, love-based belief).

Janet M.'s brother, acting as executor of their father's will, kept for himself a valuable antique Chinese vase. Although the vase was not specifically mentioned in the will, Janet was convinced that her father intended her to have it and that her brother was fully aware of this.

Janet decided never to forgive her brother. Although she had not experienced headaches or back pain before, several weeks later she began to have splitting tension headaches on an almost daily basis. At the same time, her back began to go out at regular intervals. Something as simple as leaning over to pick up the garbage would set off a wrenching pain in her lower back that would linger for several days before clearing up.

Janet began to notice that whenever she thought about her brother and felt bitter and resentful over the vase, a headache or backache would begin soon afterward. An intelligent woman, she realized that her unforgiving attitude was hurting no one but herself. So she chose to forgive her brother unconditionally.

Within a week, her headaches had disappeared and her backache never returned.

Not all pain begins with a fear-based belief. A purely physical malfunction such as osteoarthritis or tendinitis can afflict a person whose beliefs are totally positive and optimistic. But researchers believe that at least 70 percent of all chronic pain begins in the mind. Since the genesis of pain is totally subjective, by using the appropriate mental action-steps, we can squelch it right in our mind before it has a chance to begin hurting our body.

■ THE FIGHT-OR-FLIGHT RESPONSE—OPERATING IN A CRISIS MODE

Whenever the mind perceives something as hostile, threatening, or unfriendly, the brain's hypothalamus gland triggers the fight-or-flight response. This is a hair-trigger reaction that instantly readies the body to meet any threat to our survival. The kidneys squirt adrenaline and cortisone into the bloodstream to speed up metabolism and all systems are "GO."

Our muscles fill with energy and tense for action. Every artery and arteriole in the body constricts, and blood pressure shoots up. The stomach produces a surfeit of acid that irritates the stomach lining and may cause pain. The clotting ability of platelets in the bloodstream increases. And body tissues release prostaglandin, a substance that contributes to a variety of pain-provoking conditions, including inflammation. Simultaneously, brain-wave activity speeds up, and we become hyper-alert.

This response, a legacy from primitive times, prepares us to do combat or to flee from physical danger. However, the hypothalamus gland cannot distinguish whether a feeling of fear is caused by a masked gunman or by a letter from the IRS. Whether the perceived danger is real or imagined, the hypothalamus turns on the fight-or-flight reaction. Virtually any negative feeling, in fact, will set off some level of fight-or-flight response.

A feeling of resentment won't turn on the same intensity of alarm as would a charging elephant. But any degree of negative emotion—be it anxiety, depression, envy, guilt, or helplessness—will turn on some or all of the fight-or-flight mechanisms.

Many Pain Sufferers Live Continuously in an Emergency State

According to Dr. Herbert Benson, an associate professor of medicine at Harvard Medical School, modern urban life is so filled with potentially stressful situations that many people live continuously in an emergency state. Their fight-or-flight response continues to simmer, and all their basic life support systems are poised at emergency levels.

The result: millions of Americans live with perpetually constricted arteries and tensed muscles, especially in the shoulders, neck, and back. Taut and rigid, these muscles tear at the least provocation. When that happens, they spasm. Nearby nerve endings are irritated and pain impulses arise.

Meanwhile, tense and rigid muscles in the neck and shoulders irritate nerve endings that signal release of prostaglandin in the headband area of the scalp. The prostaglandin intensifies artery constriction in the hatband area. Prostaglandin also makes nerve endings in these arteries exquisitely sensitive to pain.

The stage is now set for a splitting tension headache.

Anatomy of a Headache

In a desperate attempt to bring in more oxygen and other essential nutrients, the tightly constricted headband arteries explode into a violent dilation. As sensitive nerve-endings in the arteries are stretched, they literally scream with pain—and they transmit neural impulses that the brain experiences as a distressing headache.

Interestingly, one of aspirin's principle functions is to inhibit prostaglandin synthesis. Since prostaglandin release is an essential step in the tension headache sequence, this explains why two aspirin *will* stop most simple tension headaches.

The fight-or-flight response is also one of several possible migraine headache triggers. One fight-or-flight mechanism releases the neurotransmitter norepinephrine, which, together with calcium, induces powerful constriction and spasm in arteries lining the interior of the skull.

Starved for oxygen and other essential nutrients, these arteries rebel with an explosive dilation. As in a tension headache, sensitive nerve endings are stretched and pain impulses are transmitted to the brain.

Since prostaglandin synthesis is not involved in the migraine process, aspirin is usually ineffective in relieving a migraine headache. Instead, most migraine drugs work by blocking calcium or other substances that are essential in the migraine sequence.

Through the fight-or-flight response, psychological stress is translated into physiological changes that irritate nerve endings. In turn, the nerve endings transmit pain messages back to the brain.

Even when the fight-or-flight response is triggered, it's not too late. By learning to use the body's built-in tranquilizing powers, we have the ability to slow down our emergency state and to switch back into the calm, serene relaxation response. Through action-steps that use relaxation training, abdominal breathing, biofeedback, and therapeutic imagery, we can turn off all the pain-provoking fight-or-flight mechanisms, and in a matter of minutes, we can return to a state of stress-free ease.

We, ourselves, can kick the fight-or-flight response more swiftly and more effectively than any muscle-relaxing drug. And we can do it without a doctor's prescription and free of any adverse side effects.

■ CLOSING THE PAIN GATE TO BLOCK OUT PAIN

Pain occurs when specialized nerve receptors are pressured or irritated by changes in arteries, muscles, nerves, cartilage, bones, or organs. The nerve receptors, called nocioceptors, are sensitized by chemicals called mediators so that they register the slightest hurt. The nerve endings pick up pain patterns and transmit them by electrochemical impulses through a series of nerve-fibers to the pain gate in the dorsal horn at the base of the brain.

Virtually the entire neurological part of the pain mechanism is controlled by two neurotransmitters that operate in tandem. Norepinephrine is released by the fight-or-flight reaction in response to stress or fear-based emotions. It is a stimulant that keeps the brain aroused and alert. Its overall effect is to lower the pain threshold, making us more sensitive to pain. The higher our level of stress or anxiety, for example, the more pain impulses norepinephrine permits to travel along nerve fibers and to reach the brain.

Serotonin is a natural tranquilizer that offsets and nullifies the effect of norepinephrine. Although it, too, is initially released by the fight-or-flight response, it swiftly becomes the antagonist of norepinephrine. Whenever we experience love-based thoughts and feelings, and become calm and relaxed, serotonin is able to penetrate the blood-brain barrier, and enter the brain, and turn on the relaxation response. A sufficiency of serotonin in both body and brain restricts pain impulses from reaching the brain, and it raises our pain threshold and reduces our perception of pain.

Both norepinephrine and serotonin are obtained from amino acids in our diet. The precursor of norepinephrine is the amino acid phenylalanine, while the precursor of serotonin is the amino acid tryptophan. Poor nutrition could lead to a deficiency of one or the other. A deficiency of tryptophan increases pain, while a deficiency of phenylalanine may lead to depression.

These neurotransmitters enable pain impulses to jump across the gaps, or synapses, that exist between the separate neuron cells that form each nerve fiber. To some extent, the predominance of serotonin can help slow down pain impulses in jumping the synapses.

Why Rubbing Takes the Ouch! Out of Pain

Now all this may sound like a voyage of discovery into the realm of neurology. But, it should be increasingly apparent that chronic pain is primarily a subjective phenomenon and that the best place to beat it is in the nervous system and brain.

For example, have you ever hit your thumb with a hammer then found you could rub away the pain? No, it wasn't just your imagination. It's true. And the reason is this.

Researchers have found that two types of nerve fibers carry impulses to the pain gate and brain. Slow fibers are uninsulated fibers that carry pain impulses through the spinal cord to the pain gate. Fast fibers are insulated nerve fibers in which electrochemical impulses travel 30 times as fast as in slow fibers. These fibers primarily carry sensations of pressure. Press your skin and the sensation is carried to the brain by fast fibers.

Located in the dorsal horn at the top of the spine is a neurological "pain gate" through which pain impulses must pass to travel on to the brain. Fast-fiber input has the power to overwhelm the lower brain center that controls this pain gate. When sensory overload occurs, the brain center closes the pain gate, blocking access to slow-fiber pain impulses.

Strike your thumb with a hammer and the pain impulses travel via slow fibers on through the pain gate and into the brain, where they register as pain. But immediately you begin rubbing your thumb — or even some other part of the body—fast-fiber impulses overload the lower brain center and the pain gate is partially or fully closed. Only a relatively few pain impulses get through.

Medical science has capitalized on this phenomenon by using electrical stimulation to produce fast-fiber impulses that close the pain gate. Known as transcutaneous nerve stimulation or TENS, it consists of a portable transmitter that can be switched on at any time for pain relief.

Inhibiting Pain by Closing the Pain Gate

However, discoveries in behavioral medicine have made TENS largely unnecessary. Using mental action-steps, we ourselves can close our pain gate by overloading it with mental imagery, or with thoughts and ideas that the mind sees as being more urgent and important than experiencing pain.

For example, when winning a game is perceived as being more important than feeling pain, a player is frequently able to continue playing until the end of a football, hockey, or basketball game even though the player has a painful bone fracture. Only when the game is over does the player begin to feel pain.

This same phenomenon is utilized by several action-steps that overload the pain gate with either mental imagery or with thoughts or affirmations. When the mind gives these mental action steps priority over pain, the pain gate closes and pain impulses are blocked from reaching the brain.

Incidentally, the lower brain center that opens or closes the pain gate is actually controlled by the balance of norepinephrine and serotonin. When other messages that seem more important are jamming the lower brain center, it is serotonin that takes over and closes the pain gate.

Don't forget, too, that as you learn to close your pain gate successfully through your own efforts, your enabling effect is aroused to help you succeed.

■ ON INTO THE WORLD OF NEUROPEPTIDES

Once through the pain gate, pain impulses enter the fascinating world of neuropeptides. Consisting of a small string of amino acids, neuropeptides are communications molecules. They communicate our feelings from the brain to every part of the body.

When we generate a feeling in the brain, such as anxiety, neuropeptides swiftly communicate this emotion into chemical events that intensify our experience of pain. Receptor sites for neuropeptides exist throughout the body, especially in the digestive tract. When peptides bind to these receptors, our cells translate their message into physical action. In this way, negative emotions are expressed in the body as discomfort or pain.

The very recent discovery of neuropeptides provided scientific proof that mind and body function as a single unit and that every pain has an emotional component.

I should mention at this point that every feeling we have in our mind arises out of the thought that preceded it. Think a positive, cheerful (love-based) thought and a minute or two later you'll begin to feel cheerful and optimistic. Think a negative, fear-based thought, and you'll swiftly begin to feel gloomy and depressed.

It is neuropeptides that communicate the way you feel to every part of your body and that cause the body to react in exactly the way you feel.

Your Body Mimics the Way You Feel

If you doubt this, begin thinking about someone you know who has a better job, a more exciting spouse, a more luxurious car, and a more prestigious home than you do. In most people, envious thoughts like these swiftly provoke mixed feelings of guilt, jealousy, and resentment. The mind sees your own comfort, prestige, and security as inadequate. It becomes mildly alarmed. And it turns on low levels of the fight-or-flight response. If you continue to hold these negative thoughts, you begin to experience the physical discomfort of stress.

Once a negative thought turns on a negative feeling and triggers the fight-or-flight response, neuropeptide messengers transform the entire body into a state of "dis-ease" and discomfort. Once a negative feeling is released, it's too late to turn it around.

But every one of us has full and complete control of our thoughts. Had you slipped that thought about the other person's success off your inner video screen as soon as it had appeared, and had you replaced it with a thought about, say, a beautiful garden, your mind would not have triggered any negative emotions. You would have remained comfortable, relaxed, and at ease.

If you doubt that you have control of your thoughts, try this. Sit down and close your eyes. Now, in your mind's eye, visualize a yellow tulip. Next, switch to a scene of a snow-capped mountain peak. Then "see" a red setter on your inner video screen.

Were you able to do that? Great! That proves you have full and complete control of your thoughts. You can use any of the cognitive action-steps in this book. And you can create your own neuropeptide messengers to carry out tasks that will lower your pain.

Incidentally, our minute-to-minute thoughts arise as we perceive the world through a filter of the beliefs that we hold. When we hold fear-based beliefs, we think negative thoughts that turn on negative feelings that set off the fight-or-flight response and lead to pain. When we hold love-based beliefs, we think positive thoughts that turn on positive feelings that keep us in the relaxation response and feeling good.

The fact that you were able to control your thoughts in the previous experiment is also proof that you can replace fear-based beliefs with love-based beliefs.

The Straight-Line System Pathway

Once through the pain gate, the neural pathway forks. One fork leads to the straight-line system, the other to the reticular system.

The straight-line system pathway carries sensory information about the pain directly to the brain's cortex, the center of conscious thought. Here, pain impulses are decoded by the thalamus gland and identified as pain. They then continue on to cortical centers that decipher their location.

Other cortex centers retrieve memories of how similar pain felt in the past. Each pain memory stored in our memory banks is associated with a certain symbolic shape and color. The shapes and colors associated with past pains are matched with input from our present pain. And the shape and color of a past pain that most closely matches our present pain are transferred to our present pain.

This shape and color symbolically represents our memories of a previous pain and our expectations of how our present pain will feel and how long it will last.

Again, this may sound like science fiction. But behavioral medicine action-steps allow our right brain to communicate with, and to ascertain, the shape and color assigned to our present pain. Then, by visualizing a shape and color that are entirely dissimilar to, and incompatible with, those of our present pain, we can nullify the pain symbols and break the pain sequence.

By visualizing a new color and shape for our pain, the right brain is able to communicate these symbols to the nervous system. As a result, our memories and expectations of the pain are changed, and the amount of pain we experience is reduced.

The Reticular System Pathway

This pathway carries the emotional portion of the pain message to the reticular center for processing. Pain impulses stress the reticular center. The center responds by stimulating serotonin to become dominant over norepinephrine in the cortex. Whenever serotonin is the dominant neurotransmitter, the cortex releases endorphins.

Endorphins are brain peptides that possess morphinelike qualities. These molecules bind with opiate receptors in the brain, producing a deep level of analgesia. When sufficient endorphins are released to bind with all pain receptors, pain is no longer experienced.

While the reticular system by itself is seldom able to block out pain entirely, several simple action steps exist by which we can boost endorphin release.

The simplest and most effective action step is to take a brisk 35-minute walk. Brisk swimming or bicycling or other rhythmic exercise for a similar period is equally effective in stimulating endorphin release. For those unable to exercise, endorphin release can be significantly increased by other action-steps such as deep relaxation, positive thinking, and therapeutic imagery.

Any of these action-steps will lead to experiencing a natural euphoria, similar in every way to the effect known as "runner's high." As the endorphins block all pain receptors, a wonderful feeling of well-being and relaxation replaces pain and discomfort.

One of the body's most powerful built-in pain relievers, endorphin therapy is freely available to anyone who is willing to act.

However, a word of caution is in order: overuse of narcotic drugs can desensitize opiate receptors, rendering endorphin ineffective. Narcotics must be eliminated before endorphin-releasing action-steps will work. Too, long-term feelings of depression, anxiety, bitterness, hopelessness, unforgiveness, or anger can deplete the endorphin supply, seriously impairing a person's ability to tolerate pain.

The Body-Mind Connection

Undoubtedly, some spillover exists between the body-mind's five built-in pain-zapping powers. For instance, learning how the pain mechanism functions not only seems to empower us, but it may also spill over into the placebo effect and into endorphin release and the enabling effect. No one knows to what exact degree these inner powers may interact. The important thing is, that singly or together, they all seem to work.

Another confusing phenomenon is "referred pain." Neural impulses can distort a pain's location. For instance, a pain in the wrist could be due to a tensed muscle in the shoulder pressing on a nerve. Pain in the back of the legs is often due to pressure on a nerve in the spinal area. This is one reason why any chronic pain should be medically diagnosed.

What Exactly is Chronic Benign Pain Syndrome

Pain is a warning that something is wrong. But the longer the pain continues, the more our nerve fibers "learn" to feel pain. Eventually, our nerves can become so accustomed to registering pain that they continue to "experience" pain even when the cause of the pain no longer exists.

Like a stuck automobile horn, this kind of pain is no longer a warning. It serves no useful purpose at all. Yet chronic benign pain can continue making a shambles of a person's life.

A classic example of chronic benign pain is "phantom pain" that continues to be experienced in a limb long after the limb has been removed. For example, a person who lost a left arm may continue to feel pain in the nonexistent left arm for many years. The existence of phantom pain strongly reinforces behavioral medicine's principal that pain is primarily psychological in origin.

Chronic benign pain may also be due to a cause that cannot be detected, diagnosed, or treated by mainstream medicine.

Turn On Your Own Placebo Power

The message of this chapter is that science has already discovered how much of our pain mechanism functions and that much of it functions on a highly subjective level. Yet millions of Americans still scoff at the idea that pain is a subjective experience, and they insist on looking for "something real."

The purpose of this chapter is to dispel any skepticism regarding the power of the mind in relieving pain. We've learned that pain is primarily a function of our beliefs, thoughts, and emotions and of our neuropeptides, nerve impulses, and neurotransmitters. We've also learned how a variety of action-steps can intervene in our highly subjective pain pathways and inhibit pain from being experienced.

You don't have to remember all the details in this chapter to use this book. All you need remember is that you read Chapter 2 and understood how various action-steps could intervene in, and block, the pain process.

If that sounds feasible, then you already have faith in, and believe in, the efficacy of behavioral medicine and its action-steps. Having credibility and faith in the action-steps will increase their effectiveness for you by approximately 35 percent. That's because having faith and expectation in an action-step turns on the full force of your body's most powerful natural pain-zapper, the placebo effect.

The Healing Power of Belief

The placebo effect arises from a person's belief in a therapy rather than from the therapy or treatment itself. Through believing in a therapy, hope is aroused and the mind begins to work independently of the treatment itself.

Give a sugar pill to any group of pain sufferers and tell them it will kill their pain, and invariably 35 percent will say they feel better. When ten patients with bleeding ulcers were given a sugar pill in a British hospital, and told they were receiving powerful pain-killing drugs, seven of the patients ceased to experience pain within a few hours.

Even with pain-killing drugs, relief may not come as much from a drug's pharmaceutical actions as from a patient's belief in it.

Virtually all case histories of spontaneous remission from terminal cancer reveal that the patient possessed an extremely strong, powerful, and unswerving expectation to recover and get well.

The placebo effect of reading this chapter is to give you a similar and profound level of faith, hope, and expectancy in your ability to relieve chronic pain by using the action-steps in this book.

Hope is good medicine for pain sufferers. Hope enables you to see your pain as a challenge to be overcome rather than a helpless situation you must learn to live with for the rest of your life. Knowing this should enable you to open your mind to the possibility that you *can* learn to control your pain and eventually become pain-free.

Chapter 3

*L*ET'S *G*ET *S*TARTED

The Only Thing You Can Lose is Your Pain

Using the action-steps is much simpler than is understanding the pain process. The most successful action-steps are as simple as picturing a certain shape and color in your imagination. And if you're physically able, walking briskly (or swimming or pedalling a stationary bicycle) is one of the most effective painstoppers available.

In this book, each action-step is called a "painstopper" and bears a number for easy location.

■ THE THREE CLASSES OF PAINSTOPPERS

- Class I: *Physical Action-steps That Are Effective for Every Kind of Pain.* Examples are walking, swimming, bicycling, and antipain nutrition. These are described in Chapter 4 of this book.

- Class II: *Mental Action-steps That Are Effective for Every Kind of Pain.* Examples are relaxation, biofeedback, therapeutic imagery, and belief restructuring. These are described in Chapters 5–8 and 13.

- Class III: *Physical Action-steps That Are Effective Only for a Specific Pain or for Pain in a Certain Location.* Examples are exercise, stretches, nutrition, self-massage, or use of heat and cold. They are described in Chapters 9–12 of this book.

Chapter 9 is devoted to describing physical action-steps for relieving arthritis, Chapter 10 to physical steps for relieving headaches, and Chapter 11 to physical steps for relieving lower back pain. In Chapter 12 you will find other detailed sections describing physical action-steps for relieving abdominal pain; fibrositis; angina and claudication; heartburn; knee, foot, and leg pain; pain in the neck, shoulder, and upper back; varicose veins; and neural pain such as neuritis, herpes zoster shingles, and tic douleureux.

■ HOLISTIC STRATEGY FOR PAIN RELIEF

Since chronic pain is a whole person phenomenon, we should ideally use a whole-person approach. To build a winning strategy, I recommend using the following holistic combination of action-steps:

1. At least two Class I physical action-steps (also good for all types of pain)
2. Two or three or more Class II mental action-steps (good for all types of pain)
3. Two or three or more Class III physical action-steps (each effective for a specific pain or location).

I'm leaving it to you to select whichever physical and mental pain-stoppers seem most appropriate to your personal pain situation. Under your Class I category, try to include a form of rhythmic exercise such as brisk walking, swimming, or bicycling to stimulate endorphin release. Choose two or three or more Class II mental painstoppers, each of which works on the neural or peptide level. Finally, pick two or three or more Class III physical action-steps that seem best suited to your type of pain.

For relief of chronic pain, each painstopper should be done at least once a day.

Except for the Class I rhythmic exercise routine—which everyone should do anyway, to prevent heart disease and cancer—the Class II and III action-steps take only a few minutes each and often less than that. Once they're familiar, the entire routine can often be done in 15 to 20 minutes.

For best results, your complete painstopper routine should be practiced twice each day. However, provided you exercise for 35 minutes or more, you need take only one walk, one swim, or one bicycle session each day.

Do remember that it's vital to have your pain medically diagnosed and to have your doctor's permission before using any painstopper in this book. Smokers or people with long-term chronic pain or heart disease or diabetes need to be especially cautious.

Another reason for reading Chapter 2 is to have some idea of what you are doing before rushing in and using any of our action-steps. By using an inappropriate painstopper, you could worsen pain instead of reduce it.

So stop immediately if any action-step causes pain or seems to make your pain worse. On the other hand, you needn't abandon an exercise or stretching program because of a simple muscle ache. Usually it will heal in a day or two. If one painstopper doesn't seem to work for you, switch to another.

Virtually all action-steps are dose related. Within reason, the more regularly you practice them, the greater the benefit.

Don't Let Your Age Put You Off

Provided you observe these caveats, plan to begin as soon as possible. The longer pain impulses continue, the more the nerve fibers "learn" to feel more pain. This may explain why chronic pain can continue long after the actual cause has ceased. Too, the longer chronic pain continues, the greater the likelihood that complications can multiply. And don't let your age serve as an excuse to procrastinate.

With a single exception, people aged 65 and over have fewer headaches, backaches, and muscle and abdominal pain than people aged 18 to 24 years. According to a 1992 survey sponsored by Bristol, Myers and Company, except for joint pain, older people experience significantly less chronic pain than younger people. The survey also found that the greater the number of hassles in a person's life, the higher the stress rate and the more pain a person experiences. Working mothers, for instance, reported significantly more headaches than homemakers.

So there's nothing to lose by getting started as soon as you can. In fact, the only thing you can lose is your pain.

Chapter 4

NO PAIN—ALL GAIN: PHYSICAL STRATEGIES TO HELP YOU STOP HURTING

This chapter presents a series of physical painstoppers that are effective against all forms of chronic pain. Only Painstopper #2 is likely to produce immediate results. But when permanently incorporated into your life-style, the other action-steps should play a significant role in helping to relieve your chronic pain.

PAINSTOPPER #2
Walk Away from Pain

Carole J. had suffered from rampaging tension headaches almost every afternoon for more than three months. Aspirin helped at first, but gradually she required increasingly stronger medication. The drugs would leave Carole feeling anxious and depressed. When she began to experience dry-mouth and nausea as well, Carole finally decided that any benefit the drugs offered were not worth their devastating side effects.

A friend suggested she consult a physical therapist. Her appointment was scheduled for late afternoon, and her head was already splitting with pain. Carole's knuckles were white, and she grimaced as she lowered herself into the therapist's chair.

"How often do you walk each day?" the therapist asked.

"I can't walk at all," Carole managed to say. "Right now, every move I make jars my head and makes me dizzy with pain."

But the therapist learned that Carole was pain-free each morning.

"Walking is the best all-around natural pain reliever in existence," he told Carole. "I'd like you to get up an hour earlier each morning and take a brisk 35-minute walk before breakfast."

■ TAP INTO YOUR BODY'S PAIN-EASING POWER

The therapist explained that walking briskly for 35 minutes or more, at a pace that elevates both pulse and respiration, releases endorphin in the brain. Endorphins are the body's own natural tranquilizer and a wonderful release for negative emotions.

Once released by the pituitary gland, these tiny peptide molecules bind on to pain receptors in the brain, blocking out all, or most, sensation of pain.

"It's like tapping into the body's natural morphine supply," the therapist went on. "Endorphins suppress the emotional experience of pain, and they stabilize the emotions for the rest of the day. You have to walk, or exercise, each day to release them. But once they're released, you will feel good until bedtime. Everything may seem to get worse as you age, but it actually gets better as you exercise. Nobody who is able to exercise should cheat themselves out of one of nature's best pain relievers."

Carole was cautioned to start walking at a pace that was comfortable and to increase speed and distance gradually. Her goal was to raise her pulse and respiratory rates for 35 full minutes at a time.

Every morning at 7 A.M., she walked in a nearby park. Nothing happened for several days. Then on the sixth day she was able to walk sufficiently fast to increase the rate of her heartbeat and her breathing. Perspiration appeared on her brow and her breathing was noticeably faster. She held this pace for 35 minutes.

Right away, she felt more comfortable and cheerful than she had in months. And for the first time in more than 90 days, her regular afternoon headache failed to appear. From that day on, provided she took her brisk

35-minute walk each morning, Carole remained headache free. At the same time, the stress and tension that had plagued her life also began to disappear.

Had she been unable to walk, her therapist told her she could achieve the same result by swimming or by pedaling a stationary bicycle at the same brisk pace for 35 minutes or more.

■ EXERCISE REBALANCES BODY CHEMISTRY

Carole also learned that brisk rhythmic exercise helps reduce pain and stiffness from arthritis, backache, and many other chronic dysfunctions. Provided it can be done without discomfort, the Arthritis Foundation recommends brisk walking for both osteo- and rheumatoid arthritis sufferers. A recent study at Washington University Arthritis Center, St. Louis, confirmed that vigorous daily walks, or any comparable rhythmic exercise, reduced all forms of arthritis pain. The Arthritis Foundation suggests beginning with a daily walk of 20 minutes and gradually increasing speed and distance. Besides releasing endorphin, the exercise loosens stiff, painful joints especially during rheumatoid arthritis flare-ups. Brisk bicycling is also recommended, especially for people with arthritis in the hips or knees.

The Arthritis Foundation discovered that not only does aerobic (rhythmic) exercise turn on the body's feel-good mechanism, but it also improves strength and flexibility.

Once Carole had beaten her headaches, her therapist added a short daily weight-training workout plus a few yoga stretches to improve flexibility. His goal was to make Carole virtually immune to *any* kind of pain in the future, especially headache, arthritis, and lower back pain. The strength-training and flexibility exercises also improved Carole's ability to walk.

For proof, studies at both Tufts and Harvard universities found that 90-year-old patients with arthritis were able to improve their ability to walk after working out with weights three times each week. Working out on a rowing machine has also helped improve strength and mobility in arthritis patients.

To start walking, you need only a safe, dry place to walk (such as a shopping mall) and a good-quality pair of athletic fitness walking shoes. For bicycling, use a stationary bicycle and set the resistance to "slow" at the beginning. Adjust the seat so that the leg is almost, but not quite, straight when the pedal is at its lowest point. Keep the ball of the foot on the pedal.

If you're unable to swim, consider walking back and forth in a swimming pool immersed waist-deep in water. Use the hands as paddles to help you along. For weight training, use moderate weights at first until you can do 13 repetitions of an exercise. Then increase the weight to the next step and do as many reps as you can (a strategy that also mobilizes your enabling effect to help meet your goal). With a rowing machine, begin with 10 minutes a day and increase to 20 or more.

For swimming, indoor bicycling, or strength-building exercises, it may be more convenient to enroll at a local health spa or gym. Most spas have a physical therapist on the staff who can demonstrate stretching and weight-training exercises and who will prepare a customized exercise routine without charge. Your doctor's approval is also essential before you begin any type of exercise program.

PAINSTOPPER #3:
The One Diet That Does it All

Like many pain sufferers, taste was one of the few pleasures left in life for Ronald A. So the Florida businessman ate what he enjoyed rather than what was healthy. And like so many pain victims, Ronald became addicted to foods high in fat and sugar.

When the pain from his gout, rheumatoid arthritis, and angina became intolerable, Ronald finally enrolled at a pain clinic.

"Most Americans grew up on a diet high in sweet and fatty foods, and we associate them with love, warmth, and approval," the staff nutritionist told him. "When we eat these same foods as adults, they remind us of the love, warmth, and approval we received as children. So they feel comfortable, and we become addicted to them. But I call them 'nutritional narcotics,' not because they relieve pain but because they do the opposite. The typical American diet, high in fat and sugar, actually intensifies most forms of pain. The sooner we kick these nutritional pain traps, the better."

The nutritionist was careful to explain to Ronald that while upgrading his nutrition might not bring any dramatic pain relief, it could directly or indirectly boost the effectiveness of almost every other pain-reducing technique.

The nutritionist also warned that Ronald's diet, high in meat, fat, white flour, and sugar was not only lowering his pain threshold but could easily lead to a heart attack or cancer.

"Virtually every health advisory agency is urging Americans to cut down drastically on meat, fat, and sugar and to increase our intake of fruits, vegetables, legumes, and whole grains," the nutritionist pointed out. "The average American gets 40 percent of his or her calories from fat. That's dangerously high. For a really healthy, pain-free life-style, our total fat intake should not exceed 20 percent of calories. The way to get the fat out of our diet is to eat foods that are primarily plant based instead of animal based. Our main foods should be fruits, vegetables, whole grains, and legumes plus a few seeds and nuts, not an endless round of beef, ice cream, eggs, cheese, and white bread and pastry.

"I recommend that you cut intake of meat and fat in half," the nutritionist advised Ronald, "and that at least 80 percent of your diet consists of plant-based foods. Eat fish instead of meat, and limit dairy foods to the nonfat variety."

■ HEALTHY EATING HELPS REDUCE PAIN

Ronald was instructed to be sure to eat a generous daily amount of whole grains and starchy vegetables: "That's to help ensure that an adequate supply of the protein tryptophan reaches your brain," the nutritionist said. "Inside your brain, tryptophan becomes serotonin, a natural sedative, pain-killer, and antidepressant."

The nutritionist quoted studies in Europe showing that pain patients who received an adequate supply of tryptophan experienced the same degree of pain relief as a control group taking antidepressant drugs. Members of the tryptophan group were also free of side effects, which was not the case with those taking the antidepressants.

The nutritionist explained that inside the brain, serotonin restricts the passage of pain impulses through the pain gate and it also accelerates release of endorphin.

Tryptophan, the precursor of serotonin, is plentiful in most animal-derived foods. It takes only a small amount of meat or dairy food to supply more than enough tryptophan for pain control. The problem is that people who eat substantial amounts of meat, poultry, eggs, cheese, ice cream, and other animal-derived foods have difficulty getting sufficient tryptophan through the blood-brain barrier and into the brain. That's because animal foods contain so many other proteins that compete with tryptophan for transport into the brain that relatively little tryptophan gets through.

By contrast, in people who eat a largely plant-based (high-carbohydrate) diet, competition from other proteins is minimal. Thus carbohydrates help speed tryptophan through to the brain. Once in the brain, tryptophan breaks down into serotonin, which helps lower our susceptibility to pain. This means that the fewer animal-derived foods we eat, the less likely we are to experience pain.

To ensure an adequate supply of tryptophan to the brain, we first need to obtain tryptophan from the diet. The best and safest sources are probably plain nonfat yogurt or nonfat cottage cheese or skimmed buttermilk. Fruit-flavored yogurt should be avoided. A small amount of these foods— say, one cup per day—contains ample amounts of tryptophan. It isn't necessary to consume large amounts. Plant-based foods such as bananas, avocado, pineapple, beans, soy products, and nuts also contain appreciable amounts of tryptophan.

■ CARBOHYDRATES TO THE RESCUE

To liberate this tryptophan and make it accessible to the brain, the rest of the diet should be low in fat and high in carbohydrates. (Carbohydrates are found in plant-based foods such as fruits, vegetables, legumes, and whole grains; although white bread, white flour, and sugar are also high in carbohydrates, they should be avoided.) A diet high in carbohydrates stimulates the pancreas to release insulin, which transports tryptophan through the blood-brain barrier and into the brain.

"All animal-derived foods are high in protein, and proteins in food may contribute to other forms of pain," his nutritionist told Ronald. "For instance, foods high in the amino acid tyramine may cause artery constriction that often triggers migraine headaches or related pain in the neck or jaw. And foods high in purines are the principal cause of gout. Again, foods high in fat have been linked to the pain of angina and cancer."

The nutritionist gave Ronald a list of foods and beverages identified by various researchers as persistent pain promoters.

These are the foods and beverages on the list:

Gremlin Foods That May Worsen Chronic Pain

Bacon

Beer

Bologna

Caffeinated soft drinks

Caffeine, especially coffee

Canned ham

Cheeses, especially cheddar and other natural aged cheeses

Chocolate and chocolate milk

Corned beef

Hot Dogs

Liver and other organ meats

Marinated foods

Monosodium Glutamate and any food containing MSG, especially potato chips, frozen dinners, canned soups, instant gravies, and some seasonings

Peanut Butter

Pepperoni

Pickled foods (e.g., herring)

Processed meats

Salami

Sausage

Smoked fish or meat

Wine, especially champagne and red wines

Yeast and yeast extracts and products

■ VITAMIN DEFICIENCIES LINKED TO CHRONIC PAIN

Nutritional studies also show that many chronic pain sufferers—especially those with arthritis—show severe deficiencies in a number of essential vitamins and minerals. The stress of pain also increases consumption of most nutrients.

Millions of chronic pain victims are deficient in vitamins A, the B-complex, and vitamins C, D, and E as well as the minerals calcium, magnesium, and zinc. A deficiency of these minerals may inhibit the supply of synovial fluid in arthritic joints, preventing lubrication and making joints even stiffer. Several U.S. government surveys have also found that the average American diet supplies barely 40 percent of the body's magnesium needs. A deficiency of magnesium can cause muscle spasm, leading to angina pain or headaches and to musculoskeletal pain in the neck, shoulders, or back.

Millions of other pain sufferers have also been found deficient in vitamin C. They eat almost no fruits or vegetables, the primary source of vitamin C. Yet the stress of pain consumes significant amounts of this key vitamin. It's a fairly safe assumption that any chronic pain victim who fails to eat an abundance of fruits and vegetables, or to take supplements, is deficient in vitamin C.

Various researchers have also reported that vitamin C helps lessen the pain of cancer and rheumatoid arthritis. Some years ago, Texas surgeon James Greenwood also discovered that when his patients took 1 gram of supplemental Vitamin C per day, it reduced their back pain.

The full range of B-complex vitamins is also essential to healthy functioning of the body's nervous system. A deficiency of B vitamins can cause depression, irritability, and even heart disease. Yet many refined and processed carbohydrate foods, including most white bread, have lost all their natural B vitamins and most of their fiber.

Ronald A. Beats Chronic Pain with Sound Nutrition

"You can ensure an abundance of natural, pain-fighting nutrients by eating a wide variety of fruits, vegetables, legumes, whole grains, some sunflower seeds, and a few nuts each day," the nutritionist concluded. "It supplies the brain with plenty of serotonin. And it provides all the vitamins and minerals that arthritics and other pain sufferers need. A predominantly plant-based diet also minimizes risk of ever getting heart disease, stroke, cancer, diabetes, or any other of the chronic diseases that kill most Americans."

Ronald was so impressed that he decided to change his diet immediately. Except for five servings of fish per week, and a small cup of plain, nonfat yogurt daily, his diet became exclusively plant based. (His nutrition-ist advised eating fish high in oils such as sardines, canned tuna, salmon, cod, and haddock).

Far from being dull or bland, Ronald found his new cuisine full of exciting taste experiences. His wife drew on the great culinary traditions of countries like China, India, and Japan to prepare dozens of tasty, grain-based dishes that were entirely free of meat, eggs, fat, or dairy products.

As his nutritionist had emphasized, changing to a diet low in fat and high in fiber didn't produce any immediate or dramatic pain relief. But after eating healthfully for eight weeks, Ronald realized that his angina had gradually disappeared while the pain from his gout was far less severe. Eventually, that vanished too.

Except for the fish and plain, nonfat yogurt, Ronald has become a confirmed vegetarian.

"Go back to the pain-provoking standard American diet?" he says, "Not me! This is the one diet that does it all. I still have rheumatoid arthritis but I rarely feel the pain. Me? I'm staying with a plant-based diet for the rest of my life."

PAINSTOPPER #4:
Become Your Own Pain Sleuth

It was standard practice for James L. to spend one day each week at home recovering from a crushing tension headache. He lost innumerable days each year from work. As a used car salesman, James's frequent days off disrupted his boss's schedule and cut into his own income.

"There's a pain clinic at the university," his boss finally said. "Why don't you make an appointment?"

A week later James was being interviewed at the clinic by a medical doctor who specialized in headaches.

"Whether a patient has migraine or tension headaches or backache, arthritis, or any other kind of chronic pain," the doctor said, "we urge every patient to take one simple step."

That step, he explained, was to keep a daily pain log or diary. By keeping a running record of every aspect of his pain, James would very probably see a cyclic pattern emerge. He, or his doctor, could then identify the cause of his headaches or the circumstances that triggered them.

"Keeping a pain diary is standard practice at almost all pain and headache clinics," the doctor said. "It's the best diagnostic tool in the entire field of pain medicine."

The doctor explained that chronic pain cannot be medically diagnosed, nor can it be verified by lab or clinical tests. A doctor can diagnose pain only from the patient's own description.

"It's often difficult for a doctor to recommend a treatment for something that he can't see, feel, touch, locate, or even understand," the doctor told James. "That's why keeping a careful pain diary is the best diagnostic tool for both a patient and his physician. That goes for every kind of chronic pain, not merely headaches."

James L. Tracks Down the Cause of His Pain with a Diary

James was instructed to keep a daily log and to record all events as soon as possible. First, he was to enter the season, date, day of the week, and exact time of each event that seemed to be related to, or associated with, his headaches. Using a scale of 1 to 10 he was also to record the hour-by-hour intensity of his pain, his stress and tension level, and his level of comfort and pleasure. Using the same scale, he was to note all improvements. He was also asked to note whether his pain was intermittent or continuous, throbbing or steady, limited to only one side of his head or body, and whether it occurred singly or in clusters.

He was also to observe and note the circumstances, if any, surrounding each flare-up; what medications, if any, he was taking and their results and side effects; the level of stress he experienced at work or any hassles or conflicts at home; what he ate or drank prior to pain onset; and whether the pain seemed linked to sex, exercise, caffeine, alcohol, or smoking. He was also to note his feelings prior to pain onset, such as feeling frustrated, bored, angry, anxious, or hostile. (Female pain patients are also asked to record the dates of menstruation and any apparent association with oral contraceptives.)

It took only four weeks of diary keeping before James detected a strong association with his headaches. On one day each week—a day that differed from week to week—he spent considerable time during the late afternoon discussing credit applications over the phone with a local finance company. Since potential car buyers often failed to meet the company's credit standards, James and other salesmen lost a significant number of sales. Often, James would literally beg the company to O.K. a customer's credit so that a sale could go through. When the company refused, James would feel frustrated and angry.

Record Keeping Reveals a Pain's Hidden Cause

During each of the first four weeks of log keeping, James's headache would hit soon after getting out of bed on the morning following these calls.

The next week, James avoided becoming tense and angry during the finance company call. Although he still felt frustrated, he managed to stay much calmer than during any previous session.

But next morning, his headache hit with all the weight and ferocity of a truck. The day afterward, James phoned his doctor at the clinic.

"How long were you on the phone?" the doctor asked.

"Well over an hour," James answered. "I had to use both hands to sift through the application forms and to pencil in changes."

"Did you put the phone down to do that?" the doctor asked.

"No, I kept it tucked under my chin the whole time," James explained.

"It's just a guess," the doctor surmised, "but before you make the call next week, get yourself a plug-in headset for the phone. Whatever you do, don't hold the phone in place with your chin. That could cause a crick in your neck big enough to set off a world-class headache."

James acted on the doctor's advice. During the following week's call, he wore a lightweight telephone operator's headphones and microphone while his neck remained free and relaxed.

"It seemed to relax my whole mind and body at the same time," James told his doctor later. "I didn't feel mad or upset at the finance company anymore. And, best of all, I didn't get a headache the next day."

James did not get *any* more headaches. As the weeks went by and he stayed headache-free, he realized that it was through keeping a diary that he and his doctor were able to track down the cause of his pain.

■ START KEEPING A PAIN DIARY TODAY

Obviously, you don't need your doctor's permission for this action-step. So begin today to note the same events that James was instructed to record. If after several weeks, you're unable to detect any pattern or cycle, average out the daily statistics and transfer them to a weekly or monthly chart. You can easily make one on lined or graph paper. Such a graph almost always reveals longer-term trends that help you identify the cause of your pain.

Naturally, your doctor should have diagnosed your pain first. But James's doctor could only give a diagnosis of tension headache. It often takes personal sleuthing to track down and identify the actual cause of your pain.

James felt tremendously elated by his accomplishment. Earlier, he had spent hundreds of dollars on medical consultations and on drugs that consistently failed to suppress his pain. But once he decided to act and keep a diary, it took only a few weeks of observation and record keeping, and a $50 headset, to eliminate his headaches altogether.

The elation he was experiencing, of course, was empowerment released by the body's natural pain suppressor, the enabling effect. You can learn how to unleash your own enabling effect in Painstopper #5.

PAINSTOPPER #5:
Unleash the Power of Your Enabling Effect

The *enabling effect* is the psychologist's term for the empowerment we experience whenever we learn to attribute success to our own efforts rather than to a passive therapy, such as a drug or medical treatment, worked on us by someone else.

This doesn't mean we should avoid medical treatment that is obviously necessary and successful. It does mean, however, that as soon as we take an action-step, and feel our pain diminish, we experience an upbeat feeling of aliveness and enthusiasm that propels us to tackle the next step on our way to total pain relief.

The secret to unlocking this powerful motivational force is to provide yourself with constant feedback. For example, a pain level that is gradually dropping week by week supplies all the feedback that most people need to stay motivated.

To keep your enabling effect fully turned on, whenever you adopt any action-step in this book:

1. Write down your goal.
2. Divide that goal into easily attainable subgoals.

3. The success of achieving the first subgoal will then enable you to achieve the second subgoal. And then the third, fourth, and so on.

■ PAIN-RELIEF GOALS THAT ARE EASY TO REACH

For example, when Jessica E. experienced worsening osteoarthritis pain in her knees, her doctor recommended that she lose 40 pounds.

To Jessica, losing all that weight seemed impossible. But when she divided the total 40 pounds into ten subgoals of 4 pounds each, reaching her first subgoal seemed much easier.

Jessica reached her first subgoal in just two weeks. The feedback from this first success empowered her into losing her second 4 pounds. Through attributing her success to her own efforts, her enabling effect spurred her on to lose a total of 40 pounds in just 32 weeks. (In the process, she also lost much of her knee pain.)

To maintain positive feedback, it's important to keep track of your pain level day by day and week by week. You can also reinforce your positive feedback by keeping a daily record of your levels of comfort and stress and how you feel. Your own estimate of these levels on a scale of 1 to 10 is fine.

Only by keeping a daily record of how you feel can you detect a slow but gradual drop in your pain and stress levels while your comfort level imperceptibly rises. Full instructions for keeping a pain diary are given in Painstopper #4.

Breaking up your long-term pain-relief goal into more readily attainable subgoals—and keeping a pain diary—are key to unleashing your body's enabling effect to help you fight pain.

PAINSTOPPER #6:
Stop Pain-Provoking Habits with a Rubber Band

This powerful action-step can stop any negative habit dead in its tracks and replace it with a health-fortifying habit that can help relieve your pain.

Persistent pain and cramps in the bowel area are a common symptom of diverticulosis, a condition that arises when the small pouches in the intestines become inflamed and clogged with low-residue waste. Diarrhea also often alternates with constipation. Dee Dee L. had all these uncomfortable symptoms. And her doctor—who practiced whole-person healing—had no doubts about the cause.

"Your diet contains almost zero fiber," he told Dee Dee. "All you are eating is highly refined and processed foods. These foods break down into such tiny particles that they fill up and block the pouches in your intestines. It's the inflammation that results that is causing your pain."

The doctor explained that, fortunately, a simple solution existed. All Dee Dee needed to do was to stop eating all refined and processed foods, including white flour and sugar, and switch instead to a natural diet of fresh fruits, vegetables, peas and beans, and whole grains.

"I wish I could," Dee Dee lamented. "But I live almost entirely on fast-food snacks. Every time I feel tense or uptight, which is several times a day, I head for the refrigerator. I love junk food and fatty foods and ice cream. To me they're like nutritional tranquilizers. They calm my fears and anxiety and emotions and make me feel good."

The doctor explained that Dee Dee didn't have to go on being a junk food addict. It took him only a few minutes to demonstrate a simple technique known in behavioral medicine as "stop-go switching."

Dee Dee L. Discovers the Amazing Power of Stop-Go Switching

Dee Dee agreed to give it a try. To begin, all she had to do was to wear a rubber band around her wrist.

Back home, it wasn't long before she felt nervous and tense once again. So she stood up and began to walk to the refrigerator. Then she remembered the stop-go technique. She immediately began to use step 1 of the technique. She called out "Stop! Stop! Stop!" And each time she called "Stop!" she snapped the rubber band on her wrist. This action-step brought Dee Dee to an immediate halt.

Then came step 2. Still standing motionless, she began to take five slow, deep belly breaths. With each exhalation, she asked herself one of these questions:

"What are you doing to yourself, Dee Dee?"

"Why are you doing this to yourself?"

"Is this really helping you in any way?"

"Will what you're doing relieve your chronic pain?"

"What could you do instead that would benefit your health?"

Step 3 consisted of replacing her negative intention with a positive intention or thought or act. Instead of continuing to the refrigerator, she began thinking of something more positive to do. Right away, she thought of walking briskly around the block. As she held this idea firmly in her mind, Dee Dee called out, "Go! Go! Go!" And each time she called out "Go!" she snapped the rubber band on her wrist.

The stop-go ritual provided tremendous inspiration. Dee Dee immediately went outdoors and walked around the block. When she returned, she felt better than if she had eaten the ice cream snack that had been her original intention.

Switch On Your Win Power in Under 2 Minutes

Dee Dee discovered that the stop-go technique would stop *any* kind of physical habit or even a persistent negative thought.

"It's important in step 3 never to leave your mind empty or in a void," her doctor had said. "It's not enough to merely stop something negative. You must replace it immediately with a positive act or thought."

If she couldn't think of a positive act or thought, or was at the office, she could fill the void in her mind by visualizing a pleasant scene,

"Imagine a beautiful garden or beach scene, or anything that turns on feelings of pleasure or happiness or pleasant memories," her doctor advised. "Or review a successful experience. Rehearse a pleasant or successful imagery scene beforehand so you have it ready to use. Make sure you choose a subject that will fortify your health and make you feel good."

Dee Dee found that as she used the stop-go technique, recurrences of her desire to head for the refrigerator steadily diminished. And as she witnessed her progress, her enabling effect boosted her motivation to succeed.

Once her destructive snacking had ended, Dee Dee found she enjoyed a natural diet high in fruits, vegetables, legumes, and whole grains. Within a month, her diverticulosis was no more, and her chronic pain was gone.

Whatever may be intensifying your pain, whether it's high-risk food, lack of exercise, taking unnecessary medications, failing to cope with stress, or constantly holding negative thoughts, the stop-go technique can switch you from a losing to a winning mind state in under 90 seconds.

■   WE FEEL LESS PAIN IN THE MORNING

Here's a final pain tip before we move on.

If you've noticed that your chronic pain hurts more in the afternoon and evening, it's not just your imagination. Studies using electrical pain stimulation at Chicago Medical School proved that pain tolerance in most people is 20 percent greater in the morning than in the evening.

So if you have a dental appointment or a painful treatment to face, or a task that must be done, schedule it as early in the morning as you can.

Chapter 5

EXTINGUISH PAIN WITH RELAXATION AND BIOFEEDBACK

At pain clinics all over America, mental action steps are regarded as the most powerful techniques for diminishing pain. By coping with, or even eliminating, stress, they can significantly reduce the level of all types of pain. The more of these steps you use, the more effectively they alleviate pain.

For best results, they should be learned and used in the order in which they appear in this book. Each mental action-step prepares you for, and leads you into, the next one. For instance, learning relaxation training is an essential prerequisite to learning to use biofeedback or therapeutic imagery and belief restructuring.

Many people use all four action-steps in a single session. They begin with relaxation training then flow on without pause into biofeedback and then on to therapeutic imagery and belief restructuring.

Relaxation training is a simple do-it-yourself action-step by which almost anyone can swiftly learn to transform the pain-provoking fight-or-flight response into its opposite, the pain-soothing relaxation response.

Both are involuntary body-mind states. For decades, physicians believed that only by taking a drug could we achieve any degree of control over these and similar involuntary body functions (such as our levels of blood pressure and body temperature, our rates of heartbeat and breathing, and our brainwave frequency). But in the 1960s, while investigating yoga, researchers discovered that we *could* learn to control many of our involuntary functions.

By using simple action-steps such as abdominal breathing, relaxation training, visualization, and biofeedback, almost anyone can transform muscular tension into relaxation in a matter of minutes. In the process, we can lower our blood pressure and our rates of heartbeat, respiration, and brainwaves, and we can raise the temperature of our hands and feet. We can also diminish our experience of pain by up to 50 percent or more. And as we learn to control our pain, our anxiety level drops, and this, in turn, alleviates our pain still more.

Relaxation KO's Lloyd W.'s Chronic Headaches

Thirty-five-year-old Lloyd W., an Oklahoma City insurance salesman, had suffered for years from agonizing tension headaches. Only constant medication could deaden the pain. But at a local pain clinic, therapists taught Lloyd to use relaxation training to heal his pain.

Whenever a headache would strike, Lloyd was instructed to lie down. Then, in a brief 6 seconds, he learned to release all the pent-up tension in his muscles that was causing his headache. As his crushing headache began to fade, Lloyd mentally scanned his body for any signs of lingering tension. He then used a simple visualization technique that relaxed his mind as well as his body. By this time, his headache had usually disappeared. Nowadays, Lloyd doesn't get headaches any more.

Each morning, after getting up, he practices relaxation training for 15 minutes as a prophylactic measure. Almost always, he remains calm and relaxed throughout the day. And the tension in his neck and shoulder muscles, which triggered his headaches, never has a chance to build up.

A recent survey of success rates during studies at pain and headache clinics showed that relaxation training helped 60 percent of patients with disabling chronic headaches to resume normal lives. Most people in the studies were able to reduce their pain level by an average 70 percent. Some had eliminated their pain entirely. Only a very few reported no benefit at all.

For many patients, regular relaxation training made further pain medication unnecessary. While it does not eliminate stress, relaxation training is an excellent stress-coping technique. Practiced daily, it can help prevent most types of stress-related pain. And should pain occur, it can dramatically diminish the experience of almost any kind of pain.

■ HOW RELAXATION KEEPS PAIN AT BAY

Intense pain can be felt only when our brainwave frequency is in the beta state of 14 or more cycles per second. During the fight-or-flight response, our brainwaves remain in the beta range, an active and alert mental state that frequently induces anxiety.

When we enter the relaxation state, we drop into the reverie-like alpha state in which brainwave frequency ranges from 7 to 14 cycles per second. Thus, in a truly relaxed state, intense pain cannot be experienced. Many people, in fact, are unable to experience *any* pain at all.

Obviously, the best way to beat pain is to remain in the relaxation response. As we practice relaxation training and enter the relaxation response, important physiological changes occur. The breathing rate slows from an average 15 to 22 breaths per minute to only 4 to 8. The pulse rate slows. The mind becomes clear, calm, and relaxed and free of all negative thoughts and emotions. And we drift into a delicious state of calm and serenity, thinking of nothing in particular and liberated from all outside influences. Anxiety disappears. And endorphins are released in the brain. These natural narcotics block pain receptors in the brain, preventing pain from being experienced.

Relaxation training works because body and mind are intimately connected. When body muscles are tense, the mind becomes anxious and disturbed. When body muscles are relaxed, the mind also becomes calm and relaxed. When the mind is calm and relaxed, body muscles also become relaxed.

Two simple action-steps are necessary before we can use relaxation training. First, we must learn to beat pain with abdominal breathing—this is described in Painstopper #7. Second, we must learn to identify muscular tension — this is described in Painstopper #8.

Caution: Since abdominal breathing, muscle tensing, and visualizing scenes or objects in your imagination could have possible side effects on some people, particularly on anyone with heart or lung disease, osteoporosis, or other physical dysfunction, or who may experience hallucinations or have an emotional disorder, you should obtain your doctor's approval before taking any of the action-steps in this chapter.

PAINSTOPPER #7:
Learning to Beat Pain with Abdominal Breathing

When muscles in the neck and diaphragm become contracted due to tension, they prevent the lungs from moving freely. The result is that many of us take 15–22 short, shallow breaths per minute. Breathing in this way is actually a form of hyperventilation, and it is believed to heighten anxiety.

We can easily reverse this unhealthful way of breathing by inhaling through the nose, and by taking slow, deep belly breaths. Numerous studies have demonstrated that slow, deep abdominal breathing sends messages of calm to the brain, which then turns on the relaxation response.

It takes about 3 minutes of slow deep breathing to begin to reduce the tension in muscles. After a total 5 minutes of abdominal breathing, many people experience a significant decrease in chronic pain.

Since deep, slow breathing revitalizes your entire body, I recommend that you attempt to slow respiration to 4–8 breaths per minute during all phases of relaxation training. By inhaling through the nose, you can also prevent hyperventilation.

To begin, sit on an upright chair with legs uncrossed and hands on the lap. While practicing abdominal breathing, count silently once per second.

- *Step 1:* Inhale. To the count of 4, inhale completely, filling the abdomen or bottom of the lungs first, then the middle chest, and finally the upper chest. While inhaling, place one hand on the abdomen and the other on the upper chest. You should clearly feel the abdomen expand during the first second of inhalation and the upper chest expand during the final second.

- *Step 2:* Hold the breath. Hold the breath for 4 seconds.

- *Step 3:* Exhale. Take all the time you want to exhale, although 4 seconds should be the minimum. As you exhale, empty the upper chest first and the abdomen last. As you exhale deeply, smile and relax the face muscles. With each exhalation, you can visualize tension flowing out of a leg or arm or the torso or the neck and face. Or you can imagine your exhalation carrying tension out of any muscle that feels tense.

Assuming your full inhale-exhale cycle takes 12 seconds, you will be taking only 5 breaths per minute. As you breathe, focus awareness on the breath. "Watch" the breath as it flows through your nostrils and as you exhale it.

Not everyone may be able to slow his or her breathing to 5 breaths per minute. Avoid forcing yourself to breathe at a rate that feels unnatural. Focus on breathing deeply. If you inhale only for 2 seconds, hold for 1 second, and exhale for 3 seconds, it should still serve to calm you down and keep you in the relaxed alpha brainwave state.

Naturally, you can breathe slowly only while resting. You must speed up breathing while walking or exercising. But you should continue to inhale through the nose and to take deep breaths that fill the abdomen first and the upper chest last. Breathing like this can double the amount of oxygen that reaches your cells.

Discontinue abdominal breathing if it makes you nauseous or dizzy. In this case, take two or three deep, slow breaths and then return to your usual breathing pattern for several more breaths. And so on. Take it easy, do only what you can, and avoid forcing yourself into an unnatural breathing pattern. Nonetheless, step by step, you will gradually acquire the habit of abdominal breathing.

Use abdominal breathing whenever you begin to use relaxation training. Continue to use it while relaxing for as long as it feels comfortable. However, as the body-mind becomes relaxed, demand for oxygen decreases, and breathing also becomes relaxed. During deep relaxation, many people find that while they continue to breathe in and out at the same slow pace, they take in somewhat less air. At all other times you should endeavor to fill the lungs at each breath and to breathe the abdominal way.

Once you have learned abdominal breathing, you will not need to practice this step again.

PAINSTOPPER #8:
Learning to Identify Muscular Tension

Millions of chronic pain sufferers live in such a continual state of muscle tension that they have not experienced genuine relaxation in many years. During a 1986 study at the Menninger Institute, in Topeka, Kansas, researchers Patricia Selback and Joseph Sargent discovered that many of their patients were unaware of how true relaxation felt. It took a full session of relaxation training before these patients could discern the difference between tense and relaxed states.

Before moving on to relaxation training, we must first learn to recognize exactly how each of these states feels. To get started, lie comfortably on a couch, bed, or floor rug with a low pillow under the head. Extend the arms slightly from the sides, and keep the legs straight with the feet a few inches apart.

- *Step 1:* Tense and relax the arms. Raise the left arm about 6 inches, make a fist, and tense the entire lower arm from elbow to fist. Squeeze and tense the muscles and fist as tightly as possible and hold the tension.

  Become aware of the feeling of discomfort in your left arm and hand as you continue to hold it under tension. Hold the tension for only 6 seconds. Then release it and gently lower your arm. Notice how pleasant and comfortable it feels as your left arm and hand experience immediate relaxation.

  Without pausing, repeat the same routine with the right arm and fist. As you tense the right arm, compare how it feels with your now-relaxed left arm. Hold the tension in your right arm for 6 seconds. Then release and gently lower the arm.

  Never again should you have difficulty identifying the dull ache of muscular tension and the comfortable feeling of relaxation.

- *Step 2:* Identifying tension in the face and jaw. Now that you know how tension feels, mentally scan your face looking for patches of tension. Almost everyone can identify the dull ache of muscular tension at the hinge of the jaw and in and around the eyes. Many people with chronic tension headaches experience such constant tension in the jaw that it causes their temples to ache continuously. Frequent frowning may also cause chronic tension in the forehead.

See whether you can locate additional tension in the face, mouth, forehead, and neck areas. Muscular tension in these areas is believed to be caused by anxiety.

Should you locate any areas of tension, visualize yourself (in your imagination) pouring very warm water on them to relax them. Once you have learned to recognize and identify muscle tension, you need not practice this step again.

PAINSTOPPER #9:
Relaxation Training—Nature's Prescription for Pain Relief

To make relaxation training easier to learn, I have divided it into three stages. They are:

1. Releasing tension from the muscles one by one
2. Inducing deep relaxation
3. Counting down to pain relief with a simple visualization

In practice, however, you simply flow on without pause from stage 1 into stage 2 and stage 3.

If you are unable physically to tense your muscles, use only stages 2 and 3. When performed accurately, these stages can be highly effective and successful.

Stage 1:
Releasing Tension from the Muscles, One by One

By tensing each limb or muscle group in the body as tightly as possible for 6 seconds, and then releasing, this stage burns the stored-up energy that is keeping your muscles tense and contracted.

- *Step 1:* Go to the bathroom and empty the bladder. While there, wipe the hands and face with a damp washcloth. Then go to a quiet room where you will not be disturbed and unplug the phone.

- *Step 2:* Lie down on your back on a comfortable floor rug, couch, or bed with a low pillow under your head. Keeping arms and legs straight, stretch out with arms a few inches from your sides. Begin to use abdominal breathing.

- *Step 3:* Begin by frowning as hard as you can and looking upward. Hold 6 seconds and release.

- *Step 4:* Press the tongue against the front teeth (or upper gum), screw up and tense all of the face, and close the eyes and tense the eye muscles. Tense all these tightly for 6 seconds and release.

- *Step 5:* Press the back of the head down against the pillow and arch the neck and shoulders off the couch or floor. Hold 6 seconds and release. Then roll the neck loosely from side to side several times.

- *Step 6:* Tense the neck and shoulder muscles as tightly as possible. Hold 6 seconds and release.

- *Step 7:* Tense the chest muscles as tightly as possible. Hold 6 seconds and release.

- *Step 8:* Raise the left arm about 6 inches off the floor or couch. Clench the fist tightly. Keep the arm straight. Then tightly tense the muscles all the way from the shoulder down the bicep and forearm to your fist. Hold 6 seconds, release, and gently lower your arm.

  Repeat with the right arm.

- *Step 9:* Raise the left foot 6 inches off the floor. Tense the entire limb from buttocks to toes. Curl the toes tightly if you can. Hold 6 seconds. Then release and gently lower the leg.

  Repeat with the right leg.

- *Step 10:* Next tense both buttocks simultaneously. Hold 6 seconds and release.

- *Step 11:* Tense the abdomen and back muscles. Hold 6 seconds and release.

- *Step 12:* Take 6 deep, slow breaths. With each inhalation, visualize brilliant sunshine flowing in through the soles of your feet and being drawn up the legs and spreading to every part of the body. With each exhalation, visualize any remaining tension flowing out of the body and leaving through the soles of your feet.

- *Step 13:* Roll your eyes slowly from side to side a few times, then up and down, and relax.

  You should now be in a state of deep muscle relaxation. So continue without pause into stage 2.

Stage 2:
Inducing Deep Relaxation

With physical tension gone, this step uses suggestions and visualization to deepen your relaxation. Silently repeat the suggested phrases to yourself and create a mental picture of the limb or muscle deeply relaxed. Then just let it happen. Don't try to force or hurry anything. Should a daydream intrude, slide it aside and return to your imagery.

- *Step 1:* Begin by placing your awareness on the soles of your feet. Repeat silently to yourself, "My feet feel limp and relaxed. Waves of relaxation are flowing into my feet. My feet are deeply relaxed. Relaxation is filling my feet and my legs. My feet and legs are limp and relaxed. Waves of relaxation are flowing into my thighs. My thighs feel limp and relaxed. My legs, feet, and thighs are filled with pleasure, warmth, and comfort.

  You don't have to repeat the exact words but use essentially the same message. Keep your awareness on the area you are relaxing, and picture it as limp and relaxed. Many people find it easier to visualize their legs filled with cotton and to "see" them as limp and relaxed as a piece of tired, old floor rug. Keep repeating the suggestion and imagery until the limb or muscles feel completely relaxed.

  If you prefer, you can relax one leg at a time. Should you still detect any area of tension, mentally relax it before going on.

- *Step 2:* Move your awareness next to the buttocks and tell yourself, "I feel waves of relaxation flowing into my buttocks. My buttocks feel limp and relaxed. My buttocks are filled with pleasure, warmth, and comfort."

Repeat the same suggestions and visualizations for the abdomen and back muscles, the chest and shoulders, and each arm.

- *Step 3:* Then place the awareness on the face and neck as you say, "My scalp is limp and relaxed. My forehead feels smooth and relaxed. My eyes are quiet and relaxed. My face is soft and relaxed. My mouth and tongue are limp and relaxed. My jaw is slack. My neck is limp and relaxed. I feel pleasure, warmth, and comfort everywhere in my face and neck."

The face and neck are especially important because tension appears here before appearing anywhere else in the body. By relaxing the eyes and jaw, you can often induce relaxation in other parts of the body. So double-check the eyes and jaw for any signs of lingering tension.

- *Step 4:* Finally, experience a soothing feeling of relaxation around the eyes and back into the eyes themselves. "Feel" waves of relaxation, comfort, warmth, and pleasure radiate through the scalp and forehead and down around the ears and into the back of the head and neck and into the jaw and onto the cheeks, nose, mouth, and tongue.

Your entire body should now feel soft and relaxed. So enjoy the feeling of comfort, warmth, pleasure, calmness, and well-being.

When you are ready, continue on without pause into stage 3.

Stage 3:
Countdown to Pain Relief with a Simple Visualization

You can now deepen your relaxation even further by using a simple imagery technique to relax the mind.

- *Step 1:* Begin by picturing yourself in a beautiful formal garden filled with roses, trees, and flowering shrubs. You are standing at the top of a wide stone stairway. The stairs lead down to a deep, transparent spring. So clear is the water in the spring that you can see every detail on the white sandy bottom 50 feet below.

The stairway has 20 steps. Begin slowly to descend the stairs. As you descend the first step, begin to count backwards silently from 20. At the second step say "19." Count backward on down as you descend the remaining stairs. At the count of zero, you should be standing beside the spring.

- *Step 2:* Next toss a shiny, new dime into the transparent water. Watch the coin turn, glide, dart, and flash as it slowly descends through the water. In your imagination, stay about 2 feet from the dime and watch it roll and twist as it slides down and down, deeper and deeper into the stillness and silence. After about a minute, the dime comes to rest on the white, sandy bottom.

- *Step 3:* You are now in the depths of the spring, far from telephones, traffic, noise, deadlines, or pressures of any kind. All is completely still, calm, peaceful, and relaxed.

  Say to yourself, "In my mind I feel only peace, joy, and love. My mind and body are deeply relaxed. I am completely at ease and in harmony with the world. There is nothing I have to do and nothing I need or want. I am completely content, and I am filled with pleasure, warmth, and comfort."

  Although deeply relaxed, your mind should be clear and receptive, and you should feel wide awake and aware of everything that is going on. Should any thoughts of the past or future intrude on your mind, slide them off. Keep your awareness on the here and now and continue to enjoy the present moment.

You can continue to rest and enjoy your deeply relaxed state. Or you can flow on without pause into biofeedback or into therapeutic imagery. Or you can return to normal consciousness.

Returning to Normal Consciousness

To return to normal consciousness, remain lying down. Open the eyes and move them from side to side and up and down. Wrinkle and unwrinkle the face and open and close the jaw. Roll the neck from side to side; then raise and lower the head. Move the fingers and toes; then move each limb and muscle in turn. Sit up slowly and move some more; then stand up slowly. Avoid any sudden movement.

The benefits of deep relaxation should last for several hours. For pain relief, use it twice each day, for example, before breakfast and again in late afternoon. For prophylactic use—that is, to prevent pain from recurring—one session a day is usually enough. You can also use it to get back to sleep if you wake up at night.

PAINSTOPPER #10:
Experiencing Speedy Relief from Stress and Tension

Relaxation can't be hurried or rushed. You must begin by using all three stages of the relaxation training routine. But each time you practice relaxation training, the body "learns" to relax in less and less time. Most people who are physically fit soon learn to tense every muscle in the body at the same time, a shortcut that reduces the time needed for muscle tensing to less than 15 seconds.

Then by combining visualization with a series of eight abdominal breaths, you can reach a fairly deep level of relaxation in well under 2 minutes.

Here's how to do it.

Stage 1:
Rapid Muscle Tensing

Begin abdominal breathing.

- *Step 1:* Lie down on your back on a floor rug, couch, or bed as for the full relaxation training routine. Keeping the legs straight, raise both feet about 8 inches off the floor or bed. Then raise the trunk until your head and shoulders are also about 8 inches off the floor or bed. Stretch the arms out straight in front of you and parallel to the floor.

- *Step 2:* Take a deep breath and begin to exhale. As you exhale, tense every muscle in the body at the same time. Tense the thighs, legs, and feet, and curl the toes. Tense the buttocks, back, chest, abdomen, and shoulder muscles. Make a fist with each hand and tense both arms and hands as tightly as possible. Screw up and tense the entire face, forehead, eyes, mouth, and tongue and the neck muscles.

Hold all muscles at maximum tension for 6 full seconds. Then release and lower your arms, trunk, head, and legs back to the floor or bed.

- *Step 3:* If you find this difficult, try it standing up. As soon as you have tensed and released all muscles, lie down on the rug, couch, or bed.

Whichever way you prefer to do it, most people will need to practice this routine. So plan to do it in easy stages. Tense one leg first, then both legs together. Then add the arms, then the chest, back, shoulders, buttocks, abdomen muscles, and finally the neck and face.

The next stage might be to tense and release all muscles below the waist, then to tense and release all muscles above the waist. Finally, you should be able to tense every muscle in the body at the same time for 6 seconds and release.

You'll find muscle tensing much easier if you exert yourself only while exhaling.

As soon as you finish, continue on immediately into stage 2.

Stage 2:
Mental Relaxation with Abdominal Breathing

Continue with abdominal breathing.

- *Step 1:* With the first inhalation, visualize sunshine flowing in through the soles of your feet and flowing swiftly up through the legs and body to the neck and face. During the breath-holding period, "feel" your face and neck becoming limp and relaxed. And with the exhalation, visualize all the tension flowing out of your face and leaving the body through the soles of your feet.

- *Step 2:* Use the next abdominal breath to mentally relax the right arm. Based on the following program, it should take a total of only seven deep breaths to mentally relax the entire body.

  1. Relax the face and neck.
  2. Relax the right arm.
  3. Relax the left arm.
  4. Relax the chest, shoulders, back, and abdominal muscles.
  5. Relax the buttocks.
  6. Relax the right leg and foot.
  7. Relax the left leg and foot.

  During a final deep breath silently tell yourself, "I am warm, comfortable, calm, happy, and relaxed."
  At 15 seconds per breath for eight breaths plus, say, 15 seconds for muscle tensing, the entire routine can easily be done in under $2\frac{1}{2}$ minutes.

  If you wish, you can then continue on without pause into biofeedback or therapeutic imagery and belief restructuring.

■ DEFUSING STRESS WITH RELAXATION

Should you experience stress while away from home or at work, begin using abdominal breathing. Then smile, even if you have to force yourself. The mere act of smiling automatically relaxes every muscle in the face, eyes, and mouth and induces relaxation throughout the body.

Next imagine your body hanging suspended from a hook at the top of your head. Let your shoulders drop and picture your entire spine and body hanging loose and relaxed.

Scan the body quickly for any sign of muscle tension. If you identify a tense area, briefly tense the muscles in that area for 6 seconds, and let go.

With each exhalation, picture waves of relaxation flowing down through your entire body, carrying away all tension and leaving you feeling calm and relaxed.

Look at the person or condition that triggered the stress. Forgive the person or circumstance completely and forgive yourself for perceiving a situation as unfriendly. Instead, begin to perceive it as nonthreatening.

Witness it impersonally without reacting or becoming emotionally involved. Tell yourself that by remaining calm and detached you can avoid a debilitating headache, or a flare-up of rheumatoid arthritis, or having your back go out for a week, or perhaps worse.

PAINSTOPPER #11:
Biofeedback Training—Mind over Pain

Biofeedback is an easy-to-use technique for coping with stress and for preventing, and relieving, headaches, especially migraines. Technically known as *vascular relaxation through temperature biofeedback,* it was originally developed at the Menninger Institute, by Elmer Green and other researchers. Its use has been endorsed by the Mayo Clinic, Johns Hopkins, and most leading university medical schools.

Biofeedback is based on learning to dilate arteries in the hands through the use of verbal suggestions and mental images. By silently repeating verbal suggestions, while you also make mental pictures of your hands as warm and relaxed, you are able to saturate both the left- and right-brain hemispheres with a single instruction. That instruction is to warm your hands. Because your mental pictures and verbal suggestions are unconditionally accepted by the brain, they are swiftly transformed into physiological changes.

Within a few minutes, often less, arteries and capillaries in your hands begin to dilate, allowing more blood to flow into the hands. As a result, your hands become heavier and warmer. After a few practice sessions, this effect begins to generalize, and arteries throughout the head and body begin to relax and dilate.

The benefits are numerous. Tense people usually have cold, clammy hands. That's because their fight-or-flight response is turned on and their arteries are constricted. This restricts blood flow into the hands, and the hands become clammy and cold. For our hands to be really warm, we must be in the relaxation response.

Using biofeedback takes you even deeper into relaxation than relaxation training alone. Even though you may not suffer from headaches, biofeedback can help reduce the level of almost any stress-related pain.

Biofeedback prevents headaches by keeping arteries so dilated that they are unable to constrict. As arteries in the hands and body dilate, they also draw blood away from the head. This forestalls the sudden bloating of cranial arteries with blood, an essential step in the migraine sequence. When this phase is broken, migraine headaches cannot occur.

In this way, biofeedback prevents the preliminary phase of both the migraine and tension headache process. Biofeedback has also shown a remarkable track record of relieving both migraine and tension headaches once they have begun.

Diane T. Uses Her Imagination to Beat Chronic Migraines

Diane T. was a textbook example of a migraine sufferer. Her face was pale and drawn, her shoulders were hunched, and she lived in constant dread of the next attack.

Her headaches began soon after her 26th birthday. Each year, they became more frequent and more debilitating. By the second year, she was on strong prescription drugs. Yet nothing seemed to help. Her doctor tried stronger and stronger doses. Lab tests revealed no organic reason for her headaches.

By age 31, even the most powerful narcotics were unable to subdue the hammering pain. Each month, she spent several days lying in a quiet, dark room, praying for sleep. Finally, her doctor began prescribing drugs on a "let's see if this works" basis.

"I'm literally a human guinea pig," Diane told a friend.

The friend had recently taken a course in relaxation and biofeedback training to lower her blood pressure. She told Diane that both therapies were also powerful remedies for migraine headaches. She offered to teach Diane the basics that evening.

At her friend's house that evening, Diane learned essentially the same relaxation and biofeedback methods described in this chapter.

Diane was eager to begin. Each morning, she practiced the training before going to work and again in the evening. Usually, a migraine would hit at least once a week. But it was 17 days before she experienced her first aura, the warning sign of an approaching classic migraine.

"I didn't lose a second," she phoned her friend later. "I went right into deep relaxation and then warmed my hands. By then, the aura was over. But the headache itself never began."

For the first time in years, Diane experienced a feeling of control over her headaches. Her doctor agreed to withdraw her prescription drugs.

That was nine months ago.

Occasionally, while at work, she is unable to use biofeedback and a headache begins. But as soon as she can lie down and relax, she can relieve the pain, usually in less than half an hour.

"It takes practice and commitment," Diane told her friend. "But it sure beats taking drugs. Right now, I'm using the training only once a day as a prophylactic. At most, it takes only 15 minutes."

"It's really a miracle," she added. "I used to feel a terrible burden on my husband and family. But now my whole life has changed. For me, biofeedback has been all gain and no pain."

■ STUDIES VALIDATE THE PAIN-RELIEVING POWERS OF BIOFEEDBACK

During the 1980s, a study at Chicago's Diamond Headache Clinic concluded that biofeedback helped over 70 percent of headache victims after other treatments had failed. A survey of reports from other pain and headache clinics also showed that people with classic migraine had achieved an average reduction in pain of almost 90 percent while those with common migraine had experienced a reduction of almost 80 percent.

Medical science has always regarded hand temperature as an involuntary function over which we have no personal control. Yet pain clinic studies show that, even at their first attempt, most people can learn to raise the temperature of their hands by 2 to 3 degrees within a few minutes.

These results occurred at professional biofeedback clinics equipped with state-of-the-art electronic monitoring devices. If you can obtain professional training at affordable cost, by all means get it. Otherwise, with some motivation and commitment, you can achieve surprisingly good results with the do-it-yourself version described next.

■ USING THE MIND AS A PAIN RELIEVER

Biofeedback training begins where relaxation training leaves off. Before beginning, check to see that the temperature of the room you are using is at least 72 degrees and that your hands are moderately warm to the touch. If your hands are really cold, immerse them in warm water for a couple of minutes to restore circulation; then dry them off.

To get started, carry out Painstopper #9: Relaxation Training or Painstopper #10: Experiencing Speedy Release from Tension. You should be lying on a floor rug, couch, or bed thinking of nothing in particular and enjoying your state of deep relaxation. Then, without interruption, flow on into the following steps.

- *Step 1.* In your imagination, create a pleasant, restful scene of yourself lying in the warm sun on a tropical beach. Use your imagination to experience all the sensory sights, sounds, feelings, and smells that are part of this scene.

  "See" the white sails of several sailboats out on the aquamarine sea. Overhead, a few flecks of white cloud float in the wide blue sky. "Feel" the caressing breeze and "hear" it murmuring through the palm trees. Experience the feeling of heaviness as relaxation spreads through your body.

  Feel the texture of the sunbaked sand beneath your hands and feel its warmth flowing into your fingers and palms.

- *Step 2.* Place your awareness on your hands and fingers and silently repeat these phrases.

  "Warmth is flowing into my hands."

  "My hands and fingers feel heavy and warm."

  "My hands feel quite warm."

  "My hands and fingers feel warm and relaxed."

  "My fingers are tingling with warmth."

  "My hands are glowing with warmth."

  "My hands and fingers are heavy and warm."

  Keep repeating these, or similar phrases, while you continue to picture your hands as warm and relaxed.

  Imagine that waves of heaviness, warmth, and relaxation are flowing into your hands.

- *Step 3.* Within a few minutes, the fingers of one or both hands should begin to tingle, a reliable indicator of blood vessel dilation. Immediately you detect a tingling in one hand, mentally magnify that feeling. Then, in your imagination, "transfer" it to the other hand.

  As your fingers begin to tingle, tell yourself, "My hands are heavy and tingling with warmth. The tingling in my hands is very strong. I feel calm and relaxed and warm all over."

If you have any problems, concentrate on warming only one hand, or only one finger on one hand. If you can warm a single finger, it proves that you are a good biofeedback subject.

Warming the hands is usually sufficient to abort or relieve a migraine or tension headache. During a migraine attack, artery constriction diminishes blood flow to the point where hand temperature drops by several degrees. By using relaxation and biofeedback training at the first hint of a migraine, you can often prevent hand temperature from falling. This breaks the migraine sequence, and the headache will either not occur or be much less severe.

Once you can consistently warm your hands, you can go on to include your forearms in your biofeedback routine. Later, you can use the same type of imagery and suggestion to warm your feet and legs. While warming the feet is more difficult, it has proved helpful in lowering blood pressure.

■ AFFORDABLE AIDS FOR RELAXATION AND BIOFEEDBACK

Instead of repeating your own silent, verbal suggestions, you can listen to a prerecorded audio cassette tape. Usually recorded by a hypnotist, these tapes take you swiftly into deep relaxation and then into handwarming. Alternatively, you can record your own tape. One advantage of listening to a tape is that you cannot speed up, or try to rush, the relaxation process.

Two other inexpensive devices provide subtle feedback to help monitor your progress during relaxation. They are

1. A hand-held galvanic skin response (GSR) monitor that measures skin resistance and displays it as a variable audio tone.
2. An electronic digital readout thermometer that displays the temperature of your hand (or foot) in tenths of a degree.

Either, or both, of these devices provides you with instant feedback that enables you to observe subtle movements in hand temperature or relaxation level far smaller than is otherwise possible. Although neither device is essential, both can help you swiftly learn to relax and to warm your hands.

Tapes and GSR and skin temperature monitors are often advertised in health, New Age, biofeedback, headache, or hypnotist magazines and publications.

PAINSTOPPER #12:
Soothe Your Pain with Restful Music

A study that found that relaxing, soothing music could be used in place of the verbal suggestions employed in conventional relaxation and biofeedback training was reported by psychologist Janet Lapp at the 1986 meeting of the American Psychology Association.

By combining restful music with relaxation training and biofeedback imagery, participants in the study reported having fewer migraine attacks than did those in another group who used verbal suggestions. Participants listening to music also found that they could abort migraines more swiftly than could those using conventional verbal suggestions. Researchers also found that using music worked well for relieving tension headaches.

Another study, at Royal Victoria Hospital, Montreal, revealed that many patients with terminal cancer who listened regularly to classical music were able to stop taking pain-killing drugs. The study's authors found that the more a person enjoys a piece of music, the more slowly and deeply they begin to breathe and the more relaxed they become. The authors recommended that a tempo close to your heartbeat rate should provide maximum pain relief. Several similar studies have found that listening to classical or soothing music enhances the benefits of other forms of pain therapy.

Avoid any vocal or stimulating music or jazz and rock 'n roll. Choose instrumental music that is easy to listen to, such as soothing New Age music, yogic chants, classical music, or popular tunes. After having briefly tensed your muscles, lie down or sit in a chair, and continue to use mental relaxation steps as you enjoy the music.

Many libraries have music on cassette tapes that you can borrow. Listening to calming music for 30 minutes at a time while you relax is believed to break the anxiety that triggers and reinforces the fight-or-flight response. Quiet music has also been found to relax painful muscle spasm.

■ ACTION THERAPY TURNS ON ALL THE BODY'S NATURAL, BUILT-IN PAIN RELIEVERS

Using relaxation and biofeedback training provides tangible evidence that you do have mastery over your mind and body. You are no longer a helpless victim of chronic pain. Almost any degree of relaxation causes endorphin release in the brain. Using action therapy empowers you by mobilizing your enabling effect. At the same time, your placebo power is helping to boost your success by up to 35 percent. And your mental activity provides counterstimulation that helps to close your pain gate and shut off pain impulses to the brain.

Compare this powerful feeling of accomplishment with the feeling of helplessness and passivity that frequently accompanies dependency on drug medication.

Chapter 6

THERAPEUTIC IMAGERY: PAIN RELIEF FROM WITHIN

For weeks, Eric J.'s right shoulder had felt as though it were being crushed in a vise. Eric had undergone every lab test, X-ray, and scan known to modern science, but his doctor could find nothing wrong. Finally, Eric was referred to a physician who specialized in therapeutic imagery.

"What does your pain feel like?" the M.D. asked.

"Like a huge, square block of concrete crushing my shoulder," Eric told him.

"What color is your pain?" the doctor asked.

"The concrete is painted black," Eric replied.

The doctor explained that Eric could get rid of his pain by visualizing another pain symbol, and another color, that were incompatible with a black, square block. Eric was to name the first color and symbol that came into his mind.

Almost immediately, Eric's intuition supplied the answer. In his mind's eye, Eric saw a white plastic sphere. It was the same size and weight as the concrete block, and it was filled with water.

Then Eric saw a spigot on the underside of the sphere. Water was draining out. As the water flowed out of the sphere, the pressure on Eric's shoulder became less and less oppressive.

In a few minutes, the water was gone and so was the weight that was crushing Eric's shoulder. All that remained was a lightweight plastic sphere. For the first time in weeks, the pain in Eric's shoulder had lessened, and he could move his shoulder freely.

■ USING THE MIND AS A PAIN RELIEVER

Eric had just used a form of therapeutic imagery, a mental action-step that releases the awesome healing power within the body-mind. Therapeutic imagery—also known as guided imagery or creative visualization—is considered by many pain experts to be the most effective pain-relieving technique available. In a study at UCLA Medical School, headache pain was relieved in 60 percent of participants the first time they used therapeutic imagery. In another study of patients with severe chronic pain at LaCrosse Pain and Rehabilitation Center, Wisconsin, 20 percent of the participants achieved total pain relief in just four weeks.

Therapeutic imagery had proved so successful in other medical fields that it is often used in hospitals to help patients recover sooner from operations and to lessen the need for pain-killing drugs after surgery. Imagery is also widely used by sports psychologists to train athletes for the Olympics and other world-class events. Millions of other Americans use programs such as "inner golf," "inner tennis," or "inner skiing," all based on making mental pictures of winning sports techniques in your mind, and then reinforce those images with silent, verbal suggestions.

Therapeutic imagery for pain control works in the same way. You make clear, mental pictures of your desired goal, or of a proven pain-relieving technique. Then, in most visualizations, you reinforce your imagery with silent but strongly positive verbal phrases and suggestions.

This makes for a powerful combination.

By communicating in symbol language with the right brain, and in verbal language with the left brain, we create an inner dialog that bypasses the conscious mind and saturates the subconscious with our message. Since the subconscious uncritically accepts all images and suggestions fed into it, the subconscious communicates our wishes to every nerve, gland, muscle, organ, and cell in the body. Powerful inner forces then begin to work subliminally to make our goals a reality.

For pain control, imagery is used in two different ways.

Spontaneous Imagery

This was the type used by Eric earlier in this chapter. You ask yourself what your pain feels like and what color it is. The first thing that enters your mind is the answer. These become your pain object and pain color. For example, Eric's pain object was a huge square block of concrete and his pain color was black.

You then ask yourself what would nullify your pain object and what color that would be. Again, the first thing that enters your mind is the answer. These become your pain-relief object and pain-relief color. Eric's pain-relief object was a plastic sphere, and its color was white.

In your visualization, you picture your pain object and pain color and you "see" them causing your pain. You then mentally replace them with the pain-relief object and the pain-relief color. The pain-relief symbols then neutralize your pain.

Programmed Imagery

Programmed imagery is also based on replacing a pain object and pain color with a pain-relief object and a pain-relief color. The difference is that the objects and colors are chosen by intuition beforehand. And you must follow a program that you write out yourself. This means knowing precisely what you intend to do and having all images and suggestions roughed out on paper beforehand.

■ VISUALIZE YOUR PAIN AS ALREADY GONE

Key to success in programmed imagery is to use images and suggestions that portray your pain as already gone. Even though, in reality, your pain has not yet disappeared, you visualize your images, and you word your suggestions as though it has. In the same way, you phrase and visualize everything else you want to accomplish as though it were already a fact.

If you want to be pain-free, "see" yourself as pain-free *now*. Then reinforce that image by telling yourself you are entirely free of pain.

Another example: to motivate yourself to walk briskly for 5 miles each day, you would phrase your suggestions, and you would visualize yourself, as though you were already walking 5 brisk miles each day.

In therapeutic imagery, what we "see" and what we "say" is usually what we get. So whatever it is you want to happen, visualize it as already accomplished — and use your suggestions to reinforce that image.

Whether you use spontaneous or programmed imagery, results will come sooner if you use clear, graphic images and strong, positive suggestions.

How to Make Vivid, Graphic Images

At a workshop I attended, Shakti Gawain, a prominent authority on therapeutic imagery, urged us to make all mental images as detailed and realistic as possible.

"Choose scenes and symbols that bring alive your feeling of being pain-free," she told me.

In my case, I found this was best exemplified by "seeing" myself in perfect health, with a trim, athletic build, and striding along a beach without a single pain or ache anywhere in my body.

As I visualized myself walking barefoot along the beach, I used my imagination to experience sensory impressions that reinforced the emotional content of my images. For example, I experienced how good it felt to be lean, light, and free of pain. As I visualized myself striding energetically along the beach, I "felt" the grains of sand under my feet. In my imagination, I "heard" the cries of gulls circling overhead. And I "smelled" the tang of salt in the air.

Later, I visualized myself working out with weights. As I lifted a barbell at least 10 pounds heavier than any I had ever lifted in real life, I "heard" the metallic clink of the barbell and weights.

Involving all the senses in your imagery helps to bring your mental pictures alive, and it makes your visualizations far stronger and more effective.

Imagery Always Works—Even if You're Not Good at It

Don't worry if you have difficulty making strong, vivid images and holding them in your mind. What counts most is the effort you put into making your images and the degree to which you sense and experience their content.

However, watching endless hours of TV does impair our creativeness and our ability to make images. A simple way to revive your creativeness is to imagine yourself in a place you once knew well and to walk through it, reconstructing in your mind every detail of the homes, stores, and other buildings. Then go through a house you once lived in and reconstruct it room by room. If you are successful, perhaps it's because you watched less television years ago.

If you still find image making difficult, sit down with pen and paper and describe your imagery in writing. The mere act of writing invariably produces strong images in the mind. Write out your verbal suggestions as well. Even people with good imaging ability have improved their results by writing out their pain goals rather than viewing them in mental pictures.

■ HOW TO MAKE SUGGESTIONS THAT WORK

Always employ strong, positive suggestions. And if you're using programmed imagery, speak as though your pain has already vanished. Avoid using the future tense, such as, "My shoulder pain will disappear by tomorrow."

This makes a weak, vague message to give the subconscious. Instead, use the present tense and speak as though you have already succeeded.

"The pain in my shoulder has already disappeared. As the (imaginary) icebag numbs my shoulder, I no longer experience any pain at all. I feel perfectly comfortable and at ease."

Similarly, it's far better to say, "My entire body is relaxed at all times," than to say, " I will never feel tense again."

Use only positive and active words. Never say, "I would like to ———," or "I don't ———," or "I won't ———." It's far more definite and effective to say, "I am walking 5 brisk miles each day," than to say, "I would like to walk 5 brisk miles each day."

As you progress, choose phrases that express feelings and endeavor to experience these feelings as you continue making images.

You'd be expressing feelings if you said, "I am happy and delighted to be walking for 35 minutes each day. Becoming a nonsmoker has made me really proud of myself."

Repeat each suggestion at least 4 times during each imagery session and say it silently, slowly, and clearly. Say it with anticipation and enthusiasm and avoid a reticent or hesitant style.

■ HOW TO FIND YOUR PAIN OBJECT AND PAIN COLOR

Since feelings cannot be visualized, we must use a symbol and a color to represent pain and another symbol and color to represent pain relief. Each of us has our own personal symbols and colors that our right brain uses to represent pain. For example, our right brain may "see" a headache as a flat disc and its color for headaches may be purple. It may see a chest pain as a cube and its color for chest pain may be dark blue. No two people will have exactly the same symbol or color for the same type of pain.

Thus our pain imagery is exclusively our own, and it must come from our intuition. Fortunately, our nervous system is always ready to communicate this information to us in right-brain language, giving us the shape or symbol, and the color it uses to represent pain.

At this point, I should explain that, for the same pain, your intuition usually supplies one set of symbols for use with spontaneous imagery and a different set for programmed imagery. The reason? The symbols used in spontaneous imagery represent how your pain *feels* to your right brain and nervous system, whereas in programmed imagery the pain object and color are the symbols used by your right brain when it communicates with your nervous system and body. The same principles apply to your pain-relief object and pain-relief color.

■ THOUGHT-PICTURE TECHNIQUES FOR TAPPING INTO YOUR INTUITION

Here are four quick, easy, thought-picture techniques for obtaining your pain object and pain color. They are for use with programmed imagery only.

Thought-Picture Method 1: The Disappearing Cloud

Take a deep breath and exhale, relax, and close your eyes. Visualize a green lawn. Then "see" an opaque, white cloud floating on the lawn. Almost immediately, a breeze springs up and the cloud begins to drift away. As the cloud disappears, revealed on the lawn is your pain object, shape, or symbol. Beneath the object, someone has spilled some dye on the grass. The color of the dye is the color of your pain.

Thought-Picture Method 2: Seeing Behind the Closet Door

Visualize a plain indoor wall. In the wall is a closet door. In your imagination, open the closet door. Revealed inside will be your pain object, your pain shape or symbol, and your pain color.

Thought-Picture Method 3: Letting a Marker Pen Provide the Answer

Visualize yourself sitting at a table. On the table is a large sheet of white paper. In your hand you hold a black marker pen. On the paper write, and complete, the following sentence:

"My pain symbol is ———."

Do not stop but continue to write in the blank space the first word that comes into your mind.

Then, on another sheet of paper, write:

"My pain color is ———."

And write in the first color that enters your mind.

Thought-Picture Method 4: Sketching Your Pain Symbol

Sit down at a real table with a real sheet of paper and a real pen. Make a rough sketch of your body. Shade in the area that is painful and place an "X" at the location where your pain is most intense. Then draw a picture of your pain.

As you will swiftly discover, you cannot draw pain. So ask yourself, "What shape is my pain and what object does it resemble?" Make a sketch of whatever comes into your mind.

Most people sketch their pain as a wolf with bared fangs or as a snake or alligator or as a swarm of biting ants. However, it doesn't have to be alive. Whatever comes into your mind first is the answer.

Then write down and complete this sentence, "My pain color is ———."

■ HOW TO FIND YOUR PAIN-RELIEF OBJECT AND PAIN-RELIEF COLOR

To identify your pain-relief object, and your pain-relief color, ask yourself what seems most incompatible with—or the very opposite of—your pain object and your pain color.

You may not need an intuitive answer. For example, green is the contrast color to red, and white is the opposite of black, and a pyramid or sphere is incompatible with a cube.

Or you can harness your intuition to reveal your pain-relief object and pain-relief color. To do so, simply use any one of the four thought-picture methods just described for finding your pain object and pain color.

During an imagery workshop, my pain-relief object appeared as a paintbrush dripping with blue paint with which I could paint out my pain object and pain color. Another participant, who used the closet door method to find her pain-relief object and color, "saw" a sponge with which she was to sop up the pain object and the pain color. Still another participant "saw" his pain-relief object as a white knight armed with a spear who could put to flight the savage black animal that was his pain object.

Still another way to find your pain-relief object and color is described next.

■ CREATING THE RESTFUL SCENE

Picture in your mind the most relaxing, pleasant, and enjoyable scene you can think of. Perhaps it is a thatched bungalow on a tropical island beach surrounded by exotic flowers and trees. It can be a real place or one you imagine. "Hear" restful island music, "listen" to the songs of birds, "smell" the fragrance of fruits and flowers, and "experience" warm feelings of pleasure and contentment.

Once you have learned relaxation training, you'll find that merely visualizing your restful scene can take you deeply into relaxation in just 1 or 2 minutes. Thus any time you experience stress, or lose your cool, you can swiftly regain your composure by visualizing your restful scene while you breathe slowly and deeply the abdominal way.

Your restful scene can also reveal your pain-relief symbol and pain-relief color. First, picture yourself in your restful scene. Then ask yourself:

"What object do I enjoy most?"

It could be a flower, a painting, a piece of pottery, a garment, a bicycle, or even an animal. Then ask yourself:

"What is my favorite color?"

Because you will already be experiencing warmth, comfort, and pleasure, you should have no difficulty in associating with your pain-relief object and pain-relief color.

If you have absorbed this chapter so far, you should now be ready to use therapeutic imagery to control your chronic pain.

PAINSTOPPER #13:
Silence Pain with Therapeutic Imagery

To prepare for therapeutic imagery, you must first reach a state of deep relaxation by using either Painstopper #9: Relaxation Training or Painstopper #10: Experiencing Speedy Relief from Stress and Tension. If you like, you can also deepen your relaxation by using Painstopper #11: Biofeedback Training. At this point, you should be lying comfortably on a floor rug, couch, or bed, breathing slowly and deeply, and enjoying your state of deep relaxation.

Until you begin making other images, you can picture yourself breathing in your pain-relief color and breathing out your pain color. In other words, see yourself as inhaling pain relief and exhaling pain.

Throughout your imagery session, try to breathe deeply and slowly the abdominal way. Intensify your image with each breath and make it stronger and clearer.

Although no standard program exists for using therapeutic imagery, I recommend the four-stage program described here. It may take 20 minutes or so to complete the first session. But you should soon be able to finish in 15 minutes without rushing or forcing anything. For best results, practice it three times each day.

While many people experience some pain relief quite quickly, more extensive relief may take longer. So keep practicing regularly and don't give up.

Many people practice their first imagery session in bed as soon as they wake up. You can also practice pain-control imagery should you wake up during the night and be unable to return to sleep.

The four stages consist of

1. Spontaneous pain-control imagery
2. Programmed pain-control imagery
3. A pain-healing visualization
4. Visualizing yourself pain-free and in perfect health

Flow directly on from stage 1 into stage 2 and on into stages 3 and 4 without pause. Each imagery session should include all four stages.

Stage 1: Spontaneous Pain-Control Imagery

This stage requires no prior preparation.

- *Step 1*: Begin by asking yourself four standard questions. In each case, allow your intuition to reply. The answer is the first thing that comes into your mind. Here are the questions with some typical answers.

First question:	*"What does my pain feel like?"*
Intuitive answer:	*"Like an electric drill boring into my back."*
Second question:	*"What color is my pain?"*
Intuitive answer:	*"A dark pulsating red."*
Third question:	*"What would stop the drilling and relieve the pain?"*
Intuitive reply:	*"Turning off the power and pulling out the drill, then applying an icebag."*
Fourth question:	*"What color would my back be then?"*
Intuitive reply:	*"Light blue, a cool, soothing color."*

- *Step 2:* Very briefly, visualize and "feel" the pain of the drill boring into your back at the site where the pain is most intense. In the painful area surrounding the drill, "see" your flesh as a pulsating red color.

- *Step 3:* Next, visualize a hand turning off the switch supplying power to the drill and "hear" a loud click as the switch is turned off. Then, a quarter of an inch at a time, "see" and "feel" the drill being gradually withdrawn from your back.

During this visualization, reinforce the images with silent phrases or suggestions such as these.

"The drill is no longer boring into my back. I feel better already."

"As the drill is withdrawn, I feel less and less pain."

- *Step 4:* As soon as the drill is completely withdrawn, and out of your flesh, "see" and "feel" an icebag placed on the painful area. A soothing light-blue color then spreads into your flesh and replaces the pulsating red pain color.

During this step, reinforce these images with phrases or suggestions such as these:

"The ice is numbing my back. I am completely free of pain."

"The pulsating red color has gone. My back is now a soothing, pain-free blue. The blue color has liberated me from pain. I am completely pain-free and I feel wonderful."

During spontaneous imagery, the right brain often uses ugly or hostile objects, shapes, or symbols to represent the way it feels pain. Typical pain objects may be an axe, knife, sword, spear, or hammer, red-hot iron, long, rusty nail, steel trap, or crushing weight. Or you may "see" muscles in your neck or back tied into knots.

You then visualize the pain object at the location of your pain with the flesh surrounding it suffused with the pain color. Next you imagine the pain object being withdrawn slowly from your flesh, or otherwise overcome. As this happens, you "see" the pain color being displaced by the pain-relief color.

Stage 2: Programmed Pain-Control Imagery

In this stage, you visualize direct interaction between your pain object and color and your pain-relief object and color. For programmed imagery you use the pain object and color (and the pain-relief object and color) that you obtained when using one of the four thought-picture techniques described earlier in this chapter. Do *not* use the objects and colors that you obtained in stage 1.

- *Step 1:* Begin by briefly focusing your awareness on the location of your pain. Visualize your pain object located at the most painful point. The entire painful area is suffused with your pain color.

- *Step 2:* Next "see" the pain-relief object in your hand. Its color is the pain-relief color. Your hand is also bathed in the pain-relief color. The pain-relief object is radiating warmth and comfort into your hand.

  Reinforce this imagery with phrases such as "I feel cheerful, optimistic, and confident. I know that my pain object and pain color are weak and disoriented and easily overwhelmed."

- *Step 3:* In your imagination, place the pain-relief object on the painful area next to the pain object. Almost at once, the pain-relief color begins to flow into the painful area and to displace the pain color.

  Meanwhile, repeat this, or similar, phrases "My pain-relief color has replaced the pain color. I feel better already."

- *Step 4:* Visualize the pain object melting away and disappearing. As it does, the pain-relief object moves into its place and begins to radiate soothing warmth and comfort into the painful area. Soon the pain object and pain color have completely vanished.

  Only the pain-relief object and the pain-relief color are left.

  Reinforce this imagery with phrases such as these.

  "The pain color and the pain object have vanished. The pain-relief color has soothed the pain. The pain-relief object is radiating warmth and comfort into my body. I feel wonderfully relaxed, and I am completely liberated from pain."

Stage 3: A Pain-Healing Visualization

In this stage, you visualize inner healing in action and you "see" painful areas as already healed. Focus on your painful area and picture it as it was before your pain occurred. "See" it as healthy and free of inflammation. Imagine it as warm, smooth, moist, comfortable, pleasant, at ease, youthful, flexible, and resilient and in perfect health.

Visualize any red or bruised areas as already restored to health. "See" any swollen areas or joints as shrunk back to normal size and experience them being warm, soothed, and comfortable. Picture feverish areas as cool and tense areas as relaxed. Imagine any crippled joint as flexible once more.

Finally, remind yourself that just below the thin veneer of painful symptoms that masks your wellness lies the same perfect health and freedom from pain that you once enjoyed.

Phrases to go with this imagery? Suppose you have rheumatoid arthritis in the wrist. You could say:

"My wrist is completely flexible and healed. I can do everything I did with it years ago. I can play tennis, garden, or paddle a canoe just as I did when I was 20."

"The rheumatoid arthritis has completely gone. I am liberated from pain and in perfect health." (Obviously, you are not denying that you have rheumatoid arthritis. You are merely supplying your body with a blueprint to guide it to total wellness.)

Stage 4: Visualizing Yourself Pain-Free and in Perfect Health

In this stage, you send your body a strong message about your health goals and how you want to look and feel.

- *Step 1:* Begin by recalling how you looked and felt at the healthiest time in your life. Remember how easily and effortlessly you moved, how good you felt about your life, and how content, satisfied, and fulfilled you were.

- *Step 2:* Now picture yourself in this same superhealthy state, striding (or jogging) along a beach, confident that your body can fight off any disease or infection. Visualize yourself as lean, fit, suntanned, and athletic. Involve all five senses to help portray yourself in this state of perfect health.

  "Feel" the grains of sand crunch under your bare feet, "hear" the cries of gulls wheeling overhead, "see" the gentle surf cream over your toes, and "smell" the salty tang in the air. You're feeling terrific, without a trace of pain or stiffness, and every joint in your body has complete freedom of movement. You're completely healed and you can't be sick. "See" yourself laughing and feeling carefree, relaxed, and youthful and having fun.

If you prefer, visualize your own healthy scene and see yourself mountain bicycling in Utah, cross-country skiing in Colorado, playing tennis, or doing whatever else your pain may have prevented.

- *Step 3:* As you wind down your pain-control imagery, it's important to feel and express gratitude for your pain-relief and for having been healed. (Be sure to express this gratitude even if your pain still exists.) Feel deeply grateful as you repeat phrases such as "I feel comfort, pleasure, health, and happiness all over my body. I am happy and delighted and grateful to be free of pain."

- *Step 4:* Finally, congratulate yourself for having taken a completely active role in your own recovery. Tell yourself: "I feel well, optimistic, cheerful, and filled with renewed energy. As I think, feel, image, say, and believe, so I become. Every day in every way I am getting better and better."

Returning to Normal Consciousness

Take a deep breath, and as you exhale, slowly count backward from 5 to 1. Beginning with your eyes and face, slowly move each muscle and limb in turn. Then slowly sit up.

As you return to normal consciousness, remind yourself that as your images take hold, you must be prepared to do whatever it takes to make your goals happen.

■ BEFORE YOU BEGIN

While almost everyone can use therapeutic imagery safely, if you have emotional problems or emotional instability, or if you hallucinate or are schizophrenic or psychotic or prone to hysteria, or if you have any other mental or psychological dysfunction, you should have your doctor's permission before using therapeutic imagery.

Since we also frequently get what we visualize or tell ourselves, avoid any kind of imagery that pictures something detrimental to the eyes, eardrums, or any other fragile organs. Never visualize the eyes removed from the head, and do not picture a nail or knife being driven into the eyes, ears, heart, brain, or any other vital organ. However, it's perfectly all right to visualize yourself with improved sight or hearing.

Clyde T. Tries Imagery to Relieve the Pain of Spinal Arthritis

Clyde T. had had three back operations but had been unable to return to work. Then, at age 57, his back was injured in an automobile accident. Although he recovered from the accident, several doctors confirmed that he had degenerative arthritis of the spine. Constant pain and headaches made it impossible for him to stay up for more than 2 hours at a time. No medication could relieve his constant pain, and he was forced to spend most of the day in bed or reclining on a couch.

His doctor had told Clyde that therapeutic imagery might be the best hope for relieving his chronic pain. But Clyde dismissed any kind of mental action-step as "un-American" and "flaky." Finally, however, after an unusually severe bout of pain, he agreed to give it a try. After enrolling at a local pain clinic, Clyde's first step was to attend a one-day course on the anatomy of pain. As he learned that the body's pain mechanism functioned largely on the mental level, Clyde realized that therapeutic imagery really might do more to relieve his pain than any other therapy.

The following day, Clyde was taught abdominal breathing and given relaxation training. He was then introduced to therapeutic imagery. And he quickly learned to use thought-pictures to reveal his pain object and pain color for use in programmed imagery. His pain object proved to be a serpent armed with huge fangs, and his pain color was olive green. Clyde used the same thought-picture techniques to reveal his pain-relief object (a mongoose) and his pain relief color (white).

Clyde was then taught the same four-stage visualization technique described in Painstopper #13.

Clyde T. Uses Spontaneous Imagery

As he began to use stage 1, and to practice spontaneous imagery, Clyde's intuition sent him a message in right-brain language. It told him that his pain felt as if his spine were filled with molten iron and its color was a glowing cherry red.

Clyde's intuition also revealed that he could get rid of the molten iron by opening a draincock in his tailbone and allowing the red-hot metal to drain out on the ground. He could then relieve his pain by filling his spine with ice-cold water. As the water filled the hollow center of his spine, his backbone would acquire a translucent green color.

Clyde then briefly visualized his spine filled with red-hot molten iron, and he "felt" the burning pain of spinal arthritis. Next he pictured a hand opening a draincock at the bottom of his spinal column, allowing the molten iron to flow out on the ground. In his imagination, he clearly "heard" the sound of the draincock being turned and the sputter of the molten metal falling on bare earth.

Meanwhile, he silently repeated to himself, "As the molten iron drains from my spine, my pain is draining away with it. I feel much better already."

As the last drop of molten iron hit the ground between his feet, Clyde "saw" and "heard" ice-cold water splashing and hissing down into the hollow center of his spine and filling it. At the same time, Clyde pictured his spine changing to a translucent, light-green color.

"The red-hot iron that was burning my spine is completely gone," he silently repeated. "My spine feels cool and green and comfortable. The pain is gone. I am completely liberated from pain, and I feel only comfort, relaxation, and pleasure."

Clyde T. Uses Programmed Imagery

Before beginning stage 2, Clyde roughed out on paper the images and suggestions he intended to use while practicing programmed imagery.

Clyde began by focusing his awareness on the most painful area of his spine. Next to this location, he pictured his pain object, the olive-green serpent. The serpent had sunk its fangs in his spine and Clyde's entire back had turned an ugly olive-green. Clyde had been instructed to keep this visualization as brief as possible, and he held the image in his mind for only a few seconds.

As he did so, however, he repeated to himself, "I feel cheerful, optimistic, and confident. I know that my pain object and color are weak and disoriented and can be easily overwhelmed."

Swiftly, Clyde replaced the image of the serpent with a picture of his right hand. In his hand, he held a white mongoose. Almost immediately, his hand began to feel comfortable and warm and to take on the same white hue as the mongoose.

In his imagination, Clyde placed the mongoose on his painful area, next to the serpent. The mongoose immediately seized the serpent by the neck, forcing its fangs out of Clyde's spine. As the serpent's fangs were withdrawn, the white pain-relief color began to spread all over Clyde's painful back, overlaying all traces of the olive-green hue.

Clyde reinforced this imagery by silently repeating, "The serpent is dead. The pain-relief color has replaced the pain color. I feel much, much better and more comfortable."

The serpent was now dead and its body began to disappear. The friendly, white mongoose sat triumphantly next to Clyde's spine, radiating warmth and comfort into his body and bathing his back with a white, healing light.

As the serpent disappeared, Clyde silently repeated, "The serpent and the pain-color have vanished. The pain-relief color has soothed my pain. I feel the mongoose radiating warmth and comfort into my body. I feel comfortable and relaxed, and I am completely liberated from pain."

Clyde T. Uses a Pain-Healing Visualization

As he moved into stage 3 of therapeutic imagery, Clyde pictured his back as it had been before his pain occurred. He "saw" his spine as healthful, pink, flexible, and youthful and completely free of pain. His back felt cool and comfortable, and there wasn't a trace of any redness or inflammation.

"Just below this thin veneer of pain and arthritis lies the same pain-free health I once enjoyed," Clyde repeated to himself. "My back is flexible and free of pain. The arthritis is completely gone. I am liberated from pain and in perfect health."

Clyde T. Visualizes Himself as Pain-Free and in Perfect Health

For the fourth stage of his imagery, Clyde recalled how he looked and felt at the healthiest time in his life. That had been 20 years ago, before all his back problems began. He pictured himself running easily and effortlessly, and he recalled how good he felt about every aspect of his life.

"I feel comfort, pleasure, health, and happiness all over my body," he repeated to himself. "I am delighted and grateful to be free of pain. Every day in every way I'm getting better and better."

All this took place, of course, as Clyde lay recumbent on a mat on the floor. As the imagery session drew to a close, his instructor reminded Clyde that he must be prepared to do whatever it might take to make his images become a reality.

As he returned to normal consciousness, Clyde felt more relaxed, cheerful, and confident than he had in years. His pain also seemed to have lessened.

Clyde was so impressed by his single imagery session that he continued to practice therapeutic imagery for 15 minutes or longer on three occasions every day. His pain didn't disappear overnight, and he still has spinal arthritis. But 60 days after first learning how to use therapeutic imagery, Clyde estimated that his level of pain had decreased by 60 percent.

By then, he was already able to stay up for 3 to 4 hours at a time and was once again able to drive. At last report, six months later, Clyde was able to walk for half a mile without feeling pain, and he had even applied for part-time work.

For ease in learning, practice only one stage of the imagery process at a time. The more you practice, the easier it becomes to create vivid, graphic images in your mind.

Once your pain object and pain color, and your pain-relief object and pain-relief color, have been revealed for both stages 1 and 2, you can continue to use these same symbols each time you repeat Painstopper #13. This means that you can omit the initial four questions in stage 1, and you no longer need to use the thought-picture methods in preparation for stage 2. Instead, continue to visualize the same symbols and colors you used the first time around. As you become skilled in using imagery, you can repeat each visualization step 2 or 3 times or more often.

The next chapter shows how to visualize powerful pain-relieving action-steps that range from releasing endorphin to blocking pain impulses by closing your pain gate.

Chapter 7

TUNE OUT PAIN WITH PAIN-RELIEF IMAGERY

If you've ever had a throbbing toothache and then had the dentist numb the painful gum with novocaine, you know the meaning of "blessed relief." Wouldn't it be wonderful if we could induce this same pain-numbing relief into any other part of our body that hurt.

That was exactly the way Joseph C. felt whenever his rheumatoid arthritis would flare up and leave him with a hot, searing pain in his right knee. Although the pain seldom lasted more than a week, whenever it occurred, it transformed the formerly athletic 52-year-old financial analyst into a semi-invalid.

Pain medication proved almost useless. "I just wanted to curl up and die," Joseph told a friend. "That is, until a friend at work told me about therapeutic imagery. She even offered to teach me to use it."

In a single evening, Joseph learned to relax. He was then taught a special visualization technique to relieve his pain. In a short time, Joseph learned to induce a state of pain-numbing anesthesia in his right hand. Then he was shown how to induce an equally deep pain-free state in any other part of his body by rubbing it with his already anesthetized right hand.

With a little practice, Joseph found he could mentally anesthetize his arthritic knee. At first, pain relief lasted only 30 minutes. But as he continued to practice the visualization technique, Joseph was able to make the pain in his knee disappear for several hours at a time.

Joseph was both amazed and delighted. He was even more amazed to find that, eventually, he could anesthetize his knee without even going through the visualization process. As his nervous system "learned" to stop feeling pain, he was able to induce anesthesia by merely rubbing his painful knee with his right hand. He is now able to make his pain disappear whenever it occurs.

Joseph is one of thousands of former pain victims whose suffering has been relieved by a visualization process known as "glove anesthesia."

■ BLESSED RELIEF WITH THERAPEUTIC IMAGERY

Now that you know how to relax and to use therapeutic imagery, glove anesthesia is just one of several imagery techniques you can use to help relieve your chronic pain.

Therapeutic imagery works by allowing you to intervene in your mind, the ultimate controller of pain. Besides mentally inducing anesthesia, the imagery techniques that follow may enable you to relieve chronic pain by releasing endorphin, by transferring your pain elsewhere, or by switching off your pain — all without the adverse side effects of drugs.

For severe pain, you should repeat a painstopper action-step for 15 minutes 3 times each day. When they do so, many people find that after a week's practice, their pain level is reduced by one-third to one-half. And pain relief usually lasts for several hours after each session. The more you practice, the greater the pain relief you should experience, and the easier it becomes to do the imagery.

The first step in all these visualization techniques is to enter a state of deep relaxation. So eliminate all tension by using Painstopper #9: Relaxation Training. Alternatively, you may use Painstopper #10: Experiencing Speedy Relief from Tension. If you like, you may then deepen your relaxation by using Painstopper #11: Biofeedback Training. After using one or more of these powerful action-steps, you should be lying on a bed, couch, or floor rug, thinking of nothing in particular and enjoying a delicious state of carefree relaxation.

You are now ready to flow straight into any of the following painstopper techniques.

PAINSTOPPER #14:
Suppress Pain by Closing Your Pain Gate

Through visualization, we can use right-brain language to instruct our nervous system to close our pain gate and to block pain impulses from reaching the brain.

As you may recall from Chapter 2, pain messages from the body are carried to the brain along a series of "slow" nerve fibers. As these fibers funnel from all over the body into the spinal cord, they pass through a neurological "pain gate." As long as the pain gate is in the "on" or "open" position, pain impulses are able to flow on into the brain where the hypothalamus gland experiences them as pain.

Other sensations, such as those caused by rubbing or scratching the skin, create nerve impulses that travel to the brain via a parallel series of "fast" nerve fibers. These other impulses reach the pain gates, and travel on to the brain, 30 times faster than the speed at which pain impulses move.

Perceptions of rubbing and scratching and other painless sensations that travel by fast fibers are capable of overloading cells in the brainstem that control the pain gate. Counterstimulation from creative activity in the brain has a similar effect. Singly or together, these two forms of neural stimulation can overload the brain cells that control the pain gate. The result: the pain gate is partially or fully closed, and our perception of pain is reduced or even blocked out altogether.

What Kind of Brain Activity Does it Take to Close the Pain Gate?

By monitoring marksmen as they shot at targets, and athletes during moments of peak performance, researchers at the University of Maryland discovered that dramatic changes occur in a person's mental state whenever he or she focuses on some challenging physical or mental task. The study suggests that, at such moments, our right-brain hemisphere becomes dominant and it uses the symbols of right-brain language to take control of the nervous system and body. This activity—known in psychology as "being in the flow" — overloads the pain gate with counterstimulation and blocks all or most experience of pain.

We can "catch the flow" whenever we become totally concerned with some mentally engrossing task such as solving a brain-boggling puzzle. And if you enjoy challenging your mind with logic puzzles or brain teasers, or with any mathematical problem, or even a chess game, you may divert your attention from your pain to solving the problem. This competition from your brain is recognized as more important than your pain impulses. Your brainstem cells give it priority. And it overrides your pain impulses, causing your pain gate to close.

You can use this same mechanism to close your pain gate with therapeutic imagery—and you can do it without solving problems or taking up chess.

Here is all you need to do.

- *Step 1:* Visualize the shape and color of your pain. Does your pain resemble a circle, a triangle, a trapezoid, a hexagon, a square, an ellipse, or what? Whatever shape comes into your mind is the answer.

    Visualize this shape in your mind's eye. Then, in your imagination, project it out 10 feet in front of you.

    What color is your pain shape now? Whichever color you "see" is the answer.

    Fill your pain shape with this color. Then mentally change this color to red, then to blue, green, yellow, purple, orange, white, or black or to any other color you prefer. Hold each color for at least 5 seconds and experience it.

    Now change the shape of your pain. Keeping your pain shape still 10 feet out in front of you, change its shape to a triangle, a circle, a square, a pyramid, a cube, a hexagon, or any other shape you can think of.

    As you hold each shape in your mind's eye, change its color to red then to blue, green, yellow, purple, orange, black, white or any other color you may choose. Hold each color for at least 5 seconds while you experience it.

    Return to your original pain shape. Still keeping it 10 feet out in front of you, make it 20 times its original size. Then, every few seconds, change its color to red and then to blue, green, yellow, purple, orange, white, black or any other color.

Keeping the shape 20 times its original size, change your pain shape to a triangle, then to a square, a circle, a pyramid, a hexagon, a cube, or any other shape you can think of. As you visualize each new, giant shape, hold it in your mind's eye while you change its color from red to blue, green, yellow, purple, orange, white, or black. Use any other colors you like, and experience each color for at least a few seconds.

Next reduce the pain shape to one-tenth its original size. Then, step by step, change its shape and run each shape through the entire gamut of colors, just as we've been doing.

Still projecting it 10 feet out in front of you, restore the original shape to its original size. Then fill it with water. Imagine a spigot at the bottom of the shape. In your imagination, open the spigot and allow the water to run out. "Hear" the water splash onto the ground.

Then restore the original pain shape back into your mind. Finally, release all the pain shapes and colors and rest your mind for a few seconds. Next flow on without pause into step 2.

- *Step 2:* Visualize your pain gate as being closed. Visualize an electric cable. The cable carries electrical nerve impulses from your painful area into a switch. The switch is a large, old-fashioned power switch operated by a handle. Visualize a switch that is at least 18 inches high. A cable from the other end of the switch leads into your brain.

  Visualize the switch in the "on" position, allowing electrical impulses to flow through it to your brain. Visualize an engineer with his hand on the switch.

  "See" a white cloud of sensory information buzzing around the engineer and distracting him. Unable to stand the buzzing any longer, the engineer gives a gigantic heave, and with a loud clang, the switch moves into the "off " position. The buzzing stops, and the engineer is relieved. But electrical impulses are no longer able to flow through the pain gate and into the brain.

  As you "see" and "hear" the power switch closing, silently repeat these, or similar, phrases to yourself.

"My pain gate is closed. All pain impulses are blocked off. I am in a state of complete analgesia. I am pain-free and comfortable. I feel wonderful, relaxed, and terrific all over."

Since this visualization should take only a minute or so, repeat it several times.

Then return to normal consciousness.

Call this mental gymnastics if you like. But experience shows that in nine people out of ten, a single round of this visualization will influence the pain gate to close, at least partially. Even at the first attempt, most people report a decrease in pain of at least 15 percent.

Why not distract the mind with television, you ask?

Sorry! Watching TV or a sports event is actually a very passive mental activity. Watching a program that makes you laugh can often help relieve pain. But to really get control over your pain, and to turn on your enabling effect, you must actively think and exert your mind.

PAINSTOPPER #15:
Give Yourself a "Shot" of Natural Morphine

Endorphins are the body's natural pain-killers. Also called opioids because they are chemically similar to opiates or narcotics, these complex molecules work exactly like morphine or heroin. They bind on to pain receptors in the brain and block out all, or most, sensations of pain.

Within minutes, feelings of depression, anxiety, and fatigue are replaced by strongly positive feelings of energy, optimism, cheerfulness, and hope.

Unlike pharmaceutical morphine, endorphins are available to almost everyone without prescription and free of charge. To obtain them, all you need to know is how to get your pituitary gland to release them in your brain.

One way is by using Painstopper #2: Walk Away from Pain. Thirty-five minutes of brisk, rhythmic exercise will invariably release clouds of endorphin. Take a brisk walk each morning, and you're almost sure to feel good for the rest of the day.

But a combination of relaxation and visualization can also turn on the body's feel-good mechanism. Here's how it's done.

- *Step 1:* Visualize a pain meter. Visualize a gauge, similar to the gas gauge in your car. A pointer reads from 1 to 10. Actually, this is a pain meter, and it displays the intensity of your pain on a scale from 1 to 10.

  Place this imaginary pain meter at the bottom center of your inner video screen and continue to "see" it there during the remainder of your imagery. Before going on to step 2, note the reading on your pain meter.

- *Step 2:* Visualize your brain's feel-good mechanism. Use the following symbols, or similar ones, to visualize your brain's endorphins in action.

  On the left side of your inner video screen, visualize a glowing white electric bulb. On the right side, imagine a plain white wall. Sticking out from the wall are dozens of wooden or plastic pegs, each about 4 inches long. As you've probably guessed, the electric light is your pituitary gland, and the pegs symbolize pain receptors inside your brain.

  If you're not already using it, begin abdominal breathing. Focus your awareness on the bright white light. Gradually, "see" a cloud of tiny fluorescent-white specks emerging from the light. As they continue to pour out, the specks soar across the wall and settle on the pegs.

  The specks are symbols for endorphin. As you continue to watch, the endorphin clouds become so dense that they fill the top of your inner video screen. In a short time, they completely cover every peg on the wall. The entire wall is obscured by clouds of fluorescent-white specks.

  As you rest and relax and watch the ever-more-numerous endorphins, slowly and silently repeat these phrases:

  "My brain has released huge numbers of natural pain-killers. Endorphins have completely blocked the pain receptors in my brain. I no longer experience pain or depression, anxiety, or fatigue. I feel upbeat, terrific, and elated, and I am filled with energy, hope, expectation, and well-being."

  You can strengthen this imagery by repeating it one or more times.

- *Step 3:* Read your pain meter again. Look once more at your pain meter. Notice if the intensity of your pain has fallen and by how much.

After teaching this action-step to a man suffering from chronic pain caused by an unsuccessful back operation, he told me, "I still feel the pain. But it just doesn't seem important any more."

Later, we discovered that endorphin imagery would not completely relieve this man's pain. The reason? He was taking prescription narcotic pain-killers. Although the real morphine was hardly effective any more, it had completely desensitized his brain's pain receptors. Thus if you, too, are taking narcotics for your pain, this action-step may not be totally successful. If you are *not* taking narcotics, it may induce an endorphin "high" that boosts your spirits for the rest of the day.

PAINSTOPPER #16:
Numbing Your Pain with Glove Anesthesia

Glove anesthesia is a popular pain clinic imagery that can be used to relieve pain anywhere in the body provided it is localized in a compact area.

- *Step 1:* Warming your left hand. Visualize yourself sitting in a comfortable chair. On the floor on your left is an imaginary bucket of hot water. On the floor on your right is an imaginary bucket filled with frigid, icy slush, extremely cold and numbing to the touch.

  In your imagination, immerse your left hand in the hot-water bucket. "See" the water steaming. Silently repeat to yourself, "My left hand is heavy and warm. My left hand is tingling with warmth. My left hand feels very warm."

- *Step 2:* Numbing your right hand. As soon as your left hand feels warm, "see" yourself remove it from the bucket. Then visualize yourself plunging your right hand into the bucket of ice water. Immediately, you feel the intense, piercing cold, and you experience tingling and a total numbness accompanied by a loss of feeling.

As you visualize your right hand becoming numb, repeat to yourself, "My right hand is cold and numb. My right hand is tingling with freezing cold. My right hand has lost all feeling of pain."

- *Step 3:* Transfer pain-numbing cold from your right hand to your painful area. Physically place your right hand on your painful area. Using a circular motion, physically rub your hand slowly around the area of your pain. Then move it slowly back and forth across the painful area. (If you are unable to reach the painful area with your right hand, cool and use your left hand for this imagery.)

As you physically move your cold hand across the painful area, visualize yourself transferring the pain-free numbness from your right hand to the area in which your pain is located. "Feel" your painful area becoming numb and experience the pain decreasing.

If you find actual physical movement distracting, simply place your right hand on your painful area and visualize yourself moving it around and across the location of your pain. Use this same visualization if you cannot physically reach your painful area. As your hand rests on the painful area, "see" yourself transferring the numbness from your hand into the location of your pain.

As you do, silently repeat, "I have transferred the pain-numbing cold to my painful area by touching it with my cold hand. Now this area is numb with cold and free of pain. I have anesthetized my pain with numbing cold. All my pain has disappeared."

Even at their first attempt, many people experience a pain-numbing feeling in the area of their pain, and their pain begins to diminish. Should the numbness appear to fade from your hand, "see" yourself replace it in the ice-cold bucket until it is numbed once more.

Reports from a number of pain and headache clinics reveal that, even when pain medication has failed, pain relief has been quite dramatic when steps 2 and 3 are repeated several times. And the reduction in pain usually lasts for at least several hours.

Before returning to normal consciousness, visualize yourself shaking your cold hand several times to restore feeling. By practicing this action-step regularly, many people are eventually able to anesthetize pain by merely rubbing their hand over the painful area without resorting to relaxation or visualization at all.

PAINSTOPPER #17:
Changing Your Perception of How You Feel About Yourself

If we could measure pain on a scale of 1 to 10, how do you see yourself when your pain is 10, and how do you see yourself when your pain is zero?

Before you begin to visualize, sit down at a table and make a rough sketch of how you see yourself under the following three conditions.

1. *When your pain is most intense and your pain level is 10.* Mark the location of your pain with an "X" and jot down how your pain makes you feel when at its worst.

2. *When your pain level is zero and you're feeling totally pain-free and comfortable.* Picture yourself in the most pleasant and comfortable situation you can think of. Avoid including alcohol, drugs, or tobacco in your imagery although sex is fine. Jot down the feelings you would experience.

3. *When your body and mind have become exactly the way you'd like them to be.* Most people picture themselves as lean, fit, and bronzed and in superb physical condition with the body of an athlete. Jot down the feelings you might experience if you could become exactly as you'd like to be.

Now you're ready to go into deep relaxation and to begin using the imagery steps that follow. Reinforcing your imagery with suggestions or phrases is not usually necessary in this type of imagery. However, you can do so if you wish.

- *Step 1:* Visualize how you see yourself when your pain is at its worst. Briefly re-create the pain and discomfort associated with this state. How did it feel, hear, smell, or taste?

- *Step 2:* Visualize how you see yourself when your pain level is zero. How would it feel to be in the most pleasant and comfortable situation you can imagine? Again, try to enliven this picture by re-creating any sounds, smells, tastes, sights, or sensations you associate with it. Hold this picture in your mind as you experience these pleasant sensations.

- *Step 3:* Visualize yourself as you'd like to be. As you picture yourself as you'd like to be, bring the image alive with all the sensory experiences you can think of. For example, you might "see" yourself as fit and bronzed and wearing a brief swimsuit while you enjoy a swim at a resort hotel pool. You hear the hiss of water surging past your ears, you see other swimmers admiring your powerful strokes, and you feel the sun's rays warming your skin.

As you run through these visualizations, your mind will clearly perceive that being in pain is *not* the way you want to be. Your nervous system will receive a strong message that your inner life force wants you to survive and to become as fit and healthy and pain-free as possible.

Although this technique may seem simplistic, when it comes to visual imagery, what you "see" is usually what you get. Your right brain and nervous system already know how to turn off your pain. This powerful action-step could well be the motivating force that urges them to do so.

PAINSTOPPER #18:
Transfer Your Pain Elsewhere

This well-known visualization technique enables you to transfer your pain from, say, your neck to an extremity such as the sole of your right foot. You can then take a walk — either imaginary or real — and scatter the pain into the ground. Or you might transfer a headache into your right hand, clench your right fist, and throw the pain away.

Improbable as this whole thing may sound, most people are able to achieve success after just a few days of practice. One man who suffered from throbbing, hammering migraine headaches soon learned to transfer his headache pain to the sole of his right foot. The pain in his right foot was exactly the same throbbing, hammering pain he had experienced in his head. But it seemed much less severe in this new location.

He felt so relieved, in fact, that during one session, he visualized himself taking a walk. As he walked, he "saw" the pain in his foot break up and scatter into the ground. Although he still felt mildly lightheaded, he was able to get up and take a short walk. When he returned, his entire body was free of pain.

Here is how you can do the same.

- *Step 1:* Experience your pain and its location. Focus your awareness on the painful area and briefly experience the pain. For example, you might have an excruciating and pulsating migraine headache located directly behind the right eye and temple. Keep this visualization as brief as possible.

- *Step 2:* Transfer the pain to another part of your body. To do this, transfer your awareness, together with the pain, to another part of your body, such as the sole of your left foot. This action-step will mentally transfer the same excruciating and pulsating migraine pain into your foot. It may not be any less intense, but it is usually much more bearable in the new location.

  All this does take practice. At first, you may experience only a minor shift of pain. Perhaps no more than one-fourth of your pain will manifest itself in your foot while three-fourths remains in your head. Yet after a week of regular practice, most people begin to feel the pain quite intensely in the new location while the original pain area becomes increasingly pain-free.

  You can practice this technique even when you may not have any pain. Most people who practice regularly are soon able to transfer all their pain to the new location. Most people choose the sole of a foot, or a hand, as their new pain location.

  During this stage, reinforce your imagery by silently repeating phrases such as, "The sensation of throbbing pain that I experienced in my temple has now been transferred to the sole of my right foot. Now it feels much more bearable and of less importance."

- *Step 3:* Release the pain from the new location. Visualize the pain leaving the new location. For example, you could picture your pain flowing out into the air. If you have transferred pain to your foot, you could visualize yourself walking while the pain scatters into the ground. Or, if you have transferred the pain to your hand, you could "see" yourself crushing it by closing your fist and then throwing the pain away.

Provided physical movement isn't distracting, you may actually take a walk while you imagine your pain flowing into the ground. Or you can clench your fist and physically "toss" your pain away while you visualize these same actions in your mind.

You can reinforce this imagery by silently repeating phrases such as, "My foot is completely free of pain. As I walked, the pain broke up and the pieces scattered into the ground. I feel wonderful and I have total control over pain."

■ DIFFUSE THE PAIN ALL OVER YOUR BODY

Another version of this technique is to diffuse your pain mentally over a large area of your body.

Grace D. suffered from a raw, aching pain that was concentrated in a small area of the trapezium muscle on the left side of her neck. After learning to use therapeutic imagery, she was able to diffuse this pain mentally over the entire area of her body from the waist on down. This so weakened the pain that it became no more than a minor inconvenience.

Walter K., a stockbroker acquaintance of mine, used this same methodology to diffuse a pain over his entire body below the neck. He found that his pain became so trivial and unimportant that he was able to ignore it altogether.

To maximize success, I suggest visualizing your pain spread out over as large an area of your body as possible. But never include the neck or head and do not transfer pain to any location in the neck or head nor into any body organ.

■ SYMPTOM REPLACEMENT

Yet another variation of this same technique is to change the type of pain you have. One woman found that she could change the fierce, pulsating pain of a migraine headache into a dull, steady pressure. Another woman migraine sufferer learned to change her throbbing headache into a mildly tingling sensation.

No one knows exactly how the mind achieves these phenomena. Yet each technique clearly demonstrates that anyone willing to act can learn to use the mind to manage pain.

PAINSTOPPER #19:
Project Your Pain Out of Your Body

In this technique, you picture the area of your pain detached from your body.

- *Step 1:* Determine your pain's shape and dimension. Start by focusing your awareness on the location of your pain. Determine the exact shape and size of the painful area.

- *Step 2:* Detach the pain from your body. In your imagination, detach the entire painful area out of your body and project it several feet in front of you. For example, you might picture your aching back muscles detached from your body and suspended in the air about 7 feet in front of you. Be sure to visualize the empty space in your back that the muscles formerly occupied.

  Reinforce this imagery by silently repeating phrases such as, "The raw, aching muscles are gone from my back. The space they formerly occupied is now free of pain. I am happy, warm, comfortable, and free of pain."

  Or you might project a 3-inch section of painful left elbow out in front of you, leaving a gaping hole in your elbow. If you have a headache, you might remove your entire forehead, leaving a vacant space in the top of your head where your forehead used to be.

  Be sure to experience both the painful area projected out in front of you and the empty space where your pain was formerly located.

- *Step 3:* Get rid of the pain. This step provides several options for disposing of your pain.

  First, you might "see" yourself dropping the painful area into a garbage can. You can then connect the garbage can to a hot-air balloon and see it whisked skyward and away over the horizon, never to be seen again.

Second, while the painful area is still projected out in front of you, visualize it filled with ice-cold water. As it becomes numbed, watch it turn blue. Then return it back to your body. Meanwhile, repeat such phrases as, "My elbow is filled with pain-numbing cold. My elbow is relaxed and comfortable and completely free of pain."

Third, while the painful area is still projected in front of you, visualize it filled with bright, healing sunshine. Watch it becoming warm, relaxed, heavy, and pain-free. As you do, repeat phrases such as, "My elbow is filled with healing sunshine. I feel happy and comfortable. My elbow is completely healed and pain-free. I feel happy, warm, and comfortable all over."

Perhaps you can think of other ways to manipulate the painful area while it remains detached and projected out in front of you. For instance, you could magnify or shrink it, "see" it in different colors, or visualize it bathed in a soothing green light.

These are powerful visualizations, and many people experience a significant decrease in pain after using the technique half a dozen times. Besides their pain-relieving imagery, such mental exercises also help to overload the brain with sensory stimulation so that pain impulses are unable to pass through the pain gate.

PAINSTOPPER #20:
Distorting Time

Invariably, time seems to drag by at a painfully slow pace when we're hurting, while it literally flies by during a pleasant experience. The technique described here reverses the way we perceive the passage of time. In the process, it also reverses the way we perceive pain.

If you are in pain, you can speed up the passing of time by picturing yourself experiencing the most pleasurable sensations you can think of. For example, you could "see" and "experience" yourself being given a massage in a luxurious room while members of the opposite sex bring food and drink. Use anything that arouses sensations of hedonism and deep pleasure, including sex, but excluding alcohol, drugs, or tobacco. Allow yourself ample time to daydream as you fantasize a whole series of rich pleasures.

As you enjoy this mental gratification, time will begin to flash past exactly as though the pleasures were real.

Since time seems to drag when we're in pain, the slow passing of time has become associated with perceptions of pain in our minds. By the same token, when time seems to fly past, our minds are conditioned to perceive ourselves as being in a state of comfort rather than in pain. When we use imagery to make time seem to fly by, our minds perceive ourselves as being in a state of comfort rather than in pain.

■ CREATE YOUR OWN PAIN-RELIEVING IMAGERY

With a little imagination, you can create an almost endless repertoire of pain-relieving imagery techniques. You can create images and suggestions to reinforce the effects of any other action-step in this book or to boost the effects of medication or of any other treatment you may be receiving.

We must realize, though, that therapeutic imagery is only one part of a whole-person approach. It does not replace the need for exercise or nutrition or for necessary medical treatment. Yet it *can* perform wonders in enhancing their benefits.

Chapter 8

DRIVE OUT PAIN WITH POSITIVE BELIEFS

Research into cancer and immunity has confirmed that our emotions are the largest single influence on our health and our level of comfort. Every pain has an emotional component, and in every case, the emotion is negative.

Fear, resentment, anger, hostility, guilt, envy, anxiety, frustration, and disappointment are all negative emotions. Whenever we experience one of these destructive feelings, the mind recognizes it as threatening and triggers all or part of the fight-or-flight response. Pain may then manifest as musculoskeletal tension. Or the fight-or-flight response may suppress the immune system, allowing cancer cells to survive and multiply or an opportunist infection to attack and hurt the body.

Negative emotions arise when we think negative thoughts. In turn, negative thoughts arise from holding negative beliefs. So now the whole chain of cause and effect is clear. Holding negative beliefs causes us to think negative thoughts that trigger negative emotions that set off the fight-or-flight response that creates muscle tension and impairs our immunity—a deadly combination that sooner or later leads to chronic pain or illness.

■ **REPROGRAMMING BELIEFS—A NEW WEAPON AGAINST PAIN**

The opposite is also true. Holding positive beliefs causes us to think positive thoughts that trigger positive emotions such as love, joy, or compassion. The brain perceives these feelings as nonthreatening and steers the body-mind into the relaxation response in which pain and disease are virtually unknown.

Thus the underlying cause of most chronic pain lies in the type of beliefs that we hold. Your family doctor may not be aware of this. But thousands of others are, including many of the nation's most prominent psychologists, psychiatrists, neurologists, nutritionists, immunologists, rheumatologists, cardiologists, algologists, physiatrists, physical therapists, and registered nurses. The explanation is that all these health professionals are practitioners of behavioral medicine.

When health professionals of this caliber recognize that beliefs are the underlying cause of much chronic pain and illness, their conclusions are not to be scoffed at. Nowadays, belief reprogramming occupies a prominent place among the topics taught at the nation's largest annual conference on behavioral medicine.

Beliefs centered on unforgiveness are considered a prime cause of damaging emotions such as resentment and anger. So much so that workshops such as, "Forgiveness, An Essential Component in Health and Healing," or "Ways in Which Beliefs Have the Power to Change Your Body" are regularly scheduled at major conferences sponsored by organizations like the National Institute for Clinical Application of Behavioral Medicine.

■ **THE ONE BELIEF THAT CAUSES MOST PAIN**

Among the most destructive beliefs, those concerned with unforgiveness have probably led to more chronic pain, and to more cases of cancer, than any other single cause.

At some time in her early childhood, Freda K. acquired the belief that she should never forgive an injustice. She felt badly cheated when the job she thought she was next in line for was given to her boss's niece, a recent college graduate with no prior work experience.

Whenever Freda considered how unjustly she had been treated, she would begin to feel increasingly tense and uncomfortable. But she saw no reason to forgive her boss, and she continued to feel resentful month after month.

It wasn't long before Freda began to experience burning, gnawing pains in her upper abdomen. Although the pains were intermittent, they seemed to be associated with loss of appetite and loss of weight. Taking aspirin only worsened the pain. Antacids seemed to help most. Her doctor diagnosed a stomach ulcer and prescribed stronger antacids and a medication. Despite all this, the pain slowly worsened.

■ A YOUNG PSYCHOLOGIST'S PAIN-RELIEVING SECRET

Freda described her symptoms to a cousin who had recently graduated with a degree in psychology.

Without a moment's hesitation, the cousin asked Freda whom she was mad at.

"My boss, of course," Freda gasped. "How did you know? I've worked for the company over 15 years, and I was next in line for promotion to cashier. I'll never forgive my boss for giving the job to his niece instead of to me. She's just an inexperienced girl, fresh out of college. I become furious every time I think about it. Somebody's going to pay for this injustice."

"Somebody is already paying for it," the cousin told Freda, "you are!"

At first, Freda couldn't believe that it might be her unforgiveness that was responsible for the pain of her stomach ulcer.

"Then forgive your boss," her cousin suggested. "What have you got to lose except your ulcer, your pain, and all the mental garbage you're carrying around in your belief system."

Freda's cousin explained that to get rid of an inappropriate belief, you simply let go of it.

"To do it, you do it," she said. "Just plain forgive your boss—now and forever and unconditionally. You'll be amazed at how much better you'll feel. And you'll begin to feel better right away."

Her cousin also explained that Freda should let go of any other beliefs she might still have about any injustice that might have been done to her. Or that someone must be made to pay for it.

"Whether something is just or unjust depends on how we perceive it," she told Freda. "Judging and condemning your boss hasn't hurt him. You're the one who is suffering. And it's your negative beliefs, and the destructive thoughts and emotions they engender, that are the cause of your pain."

Although her cousin's words made Freda angry, she was impressed by the young psychologist's knowledge.

"I'd do anything to get rid of my ulcer and this pain," Freda told her cousin. "Can you help me to forgive my boss and to stop destroying myself with these beliefs?"

A New Positive Belief Heals Freda's Chronic Pain

In the space of 2 hours, the cousin was able to teach Freda to relax and to use a visualization technique specifically designed for restructuring beliefs.

By bedtime that night, Freda had completely forgiven her boss and she realized that injustice was merely something that existed in her mind. She felt as if a great weight had fallen from her shoulders, and she experienced a sense of lightness and liberation that she hadn't felt in months.

She woke up the next morning feeling positive and cheerful and filled with renewed energy. Her ulcer did continue to act up on occasion. But each time the pain was briefer and less intense. Her doctor told her not to worry if the pain disappeared altogether.

"Most ulcers are caused by stress," he said. "When the stress is removed, they usually heal on their own."

It was the boss himself who helped justify it all when, a few weeks later, he told Freda that the company comptroller was quitting and that he'd been grooming Freda to assume her position and to become a vice president.

That was two years ago. Freda's ulcer has long since disappeared and her pain has vanished completely.

"As soon as I experience any kind of conflict and begin to feel stressed, I completely forgive the person involved," Freda told her cousin. "Nowadays I simply witness a conflict without making any judgments and without becoming emotionally involved. Since I avoid becoming upset, I'm better able to help solve the conflict."

Freda added that she had given up judging and condemning others. And by keeping her awareness in the here and now, Freda was able to stop worrying about the future or feeling guilty about the past.

By learning to replace her pain-provoking negative beliefs with health-enhancing positive beliefs, Freda had become completely free of pain — and that even included minor headaches and muscle spasms as well as almost all emotional pain.

The therapeutic imagery technique that she used is described next.

PAINSTOPPER #21:
Keep Pain at Bay with Positive Beliefs

To replace a negative belief with a positive belief, start by "seeing" yourself in a Zen monastery in Japan. Picture yourself barefoot and sitting cross-legged on a tatami mat floor. Directly in front of you a flame is burning on a pedestal. "Smell" the flame and the incense and "hear" a temple bell and the low chanting of monks in the distance.

- *Step 1:* Destroy the negative belief that is causing your pain. On the floor to your left you see a scroll. Pick it up and unroll it. Inside, written in English, is the negative belief that is causing your pain.

   For example, it might read: "I'll never forgive my father for what he did to me."

   Hold the scroll over the flame and watch it burn. Experience the smell of burning paper.

   A bareheaded priest wearing a gray robe comes forward. In his hand is a brass bowl. You empty the ashes into the bowl and the priest withdraws.

- *Step 2:* Place a new, positive belief in your mind. On your right you see another scroll. You pick it up and unroll it. This scroll is blank. Using a thick marker pen you write on it the new belief that will end your pain and your stress.

   In this case, you might write; "I forgive my father now, completely, unconditionally, and forever. I also forgive myself for having judged him in the first place."

   It doesn't matter what your father may have done, or how bad it was. You don't have to contact him. Simply forgive him. The alternative is to continue to suffer.

Read the new belief through slowly 3 times. Absorb it and experience it.

Once more the priest appears and takes the scroll. He tells you that the new belief is etched into your memory and will remain there forever.

- *Step 3:* Keep negative beliefs from re-entering. Visualize yourself walking out of the temple and along a path to the temple gate. Guarding the gate are two warriors, each armed with a long spear.

Imagine that one of these warriors is inside your left forehead temple and the other is inside your right forehead temple. Silently say to the warriors:

"I appoint you the guardians of my thoughts and beliefs. The belief, that I would never forgive my father for what he did to me, has been cast out of my mind. If it, or any other similar belief or thought, attempts to enter my mind, plunge your spears into it immediately. Permit only positive thoughts and beliefs to enter my mind. Spear and deflate any counterproductive thought or belief that tries to get through."

■ IDENTIFYING A NEGATIVE BELIEF THAT MAY BE CAUSING YOUR PAIN

Whenever you feel tense or upset, ask yourself what you were thinking about immediately before it happened. The following clues will help you to identify thoughts and beliefs that often trigger the fight-or-flight response:

They are primarily concerned with getting and receiving.

They judge others or attack, condemn, and criticize other people.

They cause us to expect a reward for almost everything we do.

They make us feel guilty or resentful about something that happened in the past or to become worried and anxious about what may happen to us in the future.

They cause us to compare ourselves with others and to feel discontented and dissatisfied when another person appears to be more successful or to be getting more, than we are.

They cause us to be rigid and inflexible, to have strong likes and dislikes, and to hold strong opinions.

They cause us to accept, love, and approve another person only if that person meets our conditions.

They cause us to feel insecure, either financially or in relationships.

They allow us to blame others for the way we are and for what happens to us.

Feelings of Guilt May Trigger the Pain of Rheumatoid Arthritis

Years ago, Casey S. cheated on his wife and had an affair with another woman. With some bullying and manipulating, Casey was able to persuade his wife to give him a divorce. After the divorce, he married the other woman. His ex-wife, meanwhile, was unable to find work. She began taking drugs. Eventually, she drifted into poverty, became sick, and died.

When Casey found out, he felt that he was entirely to blame for his former wife's death. Day and night, he was haunted by guilt. A few months later, swelling and pain appeared in his wrists. His doctor diagnosed rheumatoid arthritis. As Casey continued to blame himself, the arthritis spread into his elbows and shoulders.

One evening, Casey and his wife listened to a talk in a New Age church. The minister said that feeling guilty was unproductive. When we experience guilt, he said, it showed we had become a completely new and different person to the person we used to be in the past.

"We can't change the past, and we can't relive what happened," the minister pointed out. "Through our guilt, we become a better person. We would not repeat the same mistake today. So continuing to experience guilt is quite inappropriate. It merely suppresses our immune system and damages our health."

Reflecting on the minister's words, Casey decided he had been punished enough by his guilt. He chose to let go of the past and to keep his awareness focused on the present. Within hours, his spirits began to soar. He felt better than he had in months. Gradually, the redness and inflammation began to leave his joints. And within a few months, most of his arthritis symptoms had disappeared.

When we examine this belief, and Freda's belief never to forgive her boss, we find that each matches up with several of the clues that identify negative beliefs. Something in our early life establishes beliefs like these.

They may have had some validity once. But they have long since outlived their usefulness. For as long as we continue to let them run our lives, they will provoke emotional and physical pain.

When holding on to a negative belief is causing stress and pain, it's time to ask yourself what purpose that belief serves. If all it is doing is making you suffer and feel bad, then you're better off without it. Surrender its ashes to the Zen priest and replace it with a positive belief that is diametrically opposite.

■ WHAT IS A POSITIVE BELIEF?

Positive beliefs are usually written as affirmations. To maximize your health, and minimize any possibility of pain, suffering, or disease, I recommend adopting some or all of the following ten groups of affirmations. As you read them through, you may realize that you hold an opposite viewpoint or belief. If you feel under constant stress, or have a chronic pain that won't go away, you may well benefit by letting go of this opposite belief and replacing it with the positive affirmation. Use the Zen temple visualization (Painstopper #21) and reprogram only one belief at a time.

■ TEN AFFIRMATIONS THAT MAY HELP REDUCE STRESS AND RELIEVE YOUR CHRONIC PAIN

Accept Everyone Unconditionally

I accept everyone the way they are without requiring them to change. I experience a profound oneness with all other people, and I refuse to see myself as separate or different. Whenever I meet another person, I look for the similarities between us, not for the differences. I see only the best in everyone, including myself, and I cease to judge, condemn, criticize, or attack another person or to gossip about him or her. To do otherwise may compromise my emotional health and lead to chronic pain.

Let Go of Worry and Guilt

I refuse to worry about the future or to feel guilty about mistakes I have made in the past. I completely let go of the past and any guilt or resentment I feel about past events. All fears regarding the future are sheer fantasy and exist only in my imagination. Moreover, when the future does arrive, it will have become the present. For this reason, I keep my awareness in the here and now. To do otherwise may compromise my emotional health and lead to chronic pain.

Let Go of Resentment and Anger

I forgive and release everyone and every circumstance that I have not forgiven — totally, unconditionally, right now, and forever. And that includes forgiving myself. Nor do I always expect to be treated with justice and fairness. I realize that these qualities exist only in my mind, and I am ready to forgive anyone whom my mind still perceives as unjust or unfair. For I recognize that unforgiveness is a major underlying cause of cancer and one of the primary causes of chronic pain.

Let Go of Envy

I recognize that I can win only when everybody wins. So I think in terms of cooperation rather than competition. To liberate myself from envy, I avoid comparing myself with others or with their possessions and accomplishments. I also avoid envy by being willing to celebrate the good and success that comes to others. And regardless of where I am, what I'm doing, whom I'm with, or how I'm feeling, I enjoy every moment of every day. Thus I always feel comfortable and free of pain.

Be Willing to Learn and Grow

What other people view as problems I now perceive as challenges and as an opportunity to learn and grow. I accept complete responsibility for everything in my life and for everything that happens to me. To believe otherwise may compromise my emotional health and lead to chronic pain.

Realize That Absolute Security Is Unattainable

I perceive that giving and receiving are the same. Whenever I give or lose something, I will receive it back several times over. I also know that absolute material security does not exist. Yet I recognize that I will always have everything I really need. Hence I always act without anticipating results and expecting a reward for my actions. I never seek fame, recognition, or praise, and I refuse to do anything to win another person's approval. This helps me avoid disappointment, another common emotional cause of chronic pain and disease.

Be Willing to Do What It Takes to Succeed

I am willing to do whatever it takes to succeed, and I never give up or give in. I am willing to step outside my comfort zone, and I am not intimidated by minor discomfort or inconvenience or by mental or physical exertion. I always act as if failure is impossible. Hence my mind has no room for negative beliefs that may provoke pain.

Let Go of Fear

I can heal my pain — and I will! For healing is to let go of all fear-based beliefs. My birthright is to be completely free of pain and in perfect health. So every day, in every way, I am feeling better and better. To do otherwise may compromise my health and lead to chronic pain.

Let Go of Hopelessness and Negativity

I think and act positively every moment of the day. I am always hopeful, cheerful, optimistic, and positive. I expect good things to come my way today, tomorrow, and always. I recognize that to exist is bliss, to be here is joy, and to be alive is sheer happiness. Joy, happiness, and bliss are also my birthright; I can enjoy them endlessly unless I permit a fear-based belief or thought to enter my mind.

Let Contentment and Inner Peace Drive Out Pain

I cease craving superficial excitement or stimulation. I am content to be wherever I am right now. I realize that I always have whatever I need to enjoy the present moment. I also recognize that lasting happiness, fulfillment, and satisfaction arise only from feeling content and not from things that I do, buy, eat, or drink. Hence I do and acquire only things that help to deepen and maintain my inner peace. I am also careful to make choices and decisions only when I am centered, calm, and relaxed. When I feel content and at ease, and my body-mind is calm and serene, my wellness soars and I am unable to experience pain.

■ HELPING TO K.O. PAIN-CAUSING BELIEFS

When you actually analyze the cause of stress in your life, you will find that most is due to perceiving the world through beliefs that are the opposite of the beliefs just listed. By changing over to positive beliefs, we can rid ourselves of most of the stress in our lives. And since most pain is stress-related, belief reprogramming is often the most successful way to relieve ourselves from chronic pain.

Select the belief that you consider is most responsible for causing stress and pain in your life. Then use Painstopper #21 to reprogram this same belief. Use it each day for one week. Once you feel confident that this belief has been replaced, select what you consider is your second most destructive belief. Reprogram that in the same way. Keep reprogramming one negative belief each week.

Besides using the Zen temple visualization, you can repeat the new, positive affirmation to yourself at intervals during the day.

You will find it all easier to do if you focus on only a single affirmation at a time. For instance, focus on the single affirmation, "I accept everyone the way they are without requiring them to change," rather than on all four of the affirmations listed under "Accept Everyone Unconditionally."

Above all, don't put off working on your beliefs because the pain may be in your head or your back. The underlying cause of most back pain, as well as most headaches, is muscular tension caused by stress that arises from holding inappropriate beliefs. As we'll find in the next section, physical action-steps also play a major role in pain relief. But for best results, we need to employ a whole-person approach, combining both mental and physical action-steps to provide whole-person healing.

Chapter 9

NATURAL WAYS TO RELIEVE ARTHRITIS PAIN

We hear a lot about the savage pain caused by AIDS, terminal cancer, herniated spinal discs, cluster headaches, or the dreaded tic douleureux. Then there's causalgia: chronic pain due to injuries or surgery. Yet none of these anguishing conditions ranks as a very common cause of chronic pain. The great majority of persistent pain is due to arthritis and headaches, and to pain in the lower back, with knee, neck, shoulder, abdominal, and nerve pain running close behind.

Each of the physical action-steps in the following chapters may help to relieve chronic pain associated with these more common dysfunctions. However, this class of action-step is effective only for a specific pain or for a pain in a certain location.

For this reason, these physical action-steps should be used only for pain that has been medically diagnosed, and they should be used only with your doctor's approval.

The case histories in the following chapters involve people who used only physical action-steps to relieve chronic pain. Directly or indirectly, however, unresolved emotional stress remains the underlying cause of most chronic pain. And the experience of pain remains primarily a mental process. In many of our case histories, swifter and more complete pain relief might have occurred had Class I and II action-steps been used in addition to create a whole-person approach. A whole-person approach allows pain to be alleviated on both the physical and psychological levels simultaneously.

Wilma H. had suffered permanent damage to her spinal vertebrae from rheumatoid arthritis, her doctor said. He told her that she would probably never walk without pain again.

"To me that sounded like a death sentence," Wilma told a friend. "I just have to be doing something in my garden, or enjoying beautiful scenery in a park or in the country. I'm an active person and I don't enjoy being driven around. I wanted to walk."

So Wilma made a list of reasons for living and another list for dying. She found there was not a single reason to die, but she had dozens of reasons for living.

"My doctor scoffed when I mentioned therapeutic imagery," she said. "But his negative prognosis was a powerful form of imagery. By telling me I would never walk again without pain, he placed a self-fulfilling prophecy in my mind."

Since Wilma didn't have any reason for dying, or for being crippled with pain, she decided to prove her doctor wrong.

"I absolutely refused to give up," she explained.

Wilma began to hobble around with a cane. She joined an exercise program for people with arthritis. Her instructor introduced her to sound nutrition. She replaced all flesh foods with oily fish like tuna or mackerel. She learned to relax. And she began sleeping on top of her bed in a down sleeping bag.

Ninety days later, Wilma was able to walk half a mile at a time—and with almost no hint of pain.

She felt so buoyed by her success that she became a volunteer and began counseling people with terminal cancer. She saw men and women who were in far greater pain than she had ever been.

Wilma's life became so busy that she had no time to focus on her pain. She continued to improve, and she had never felt more cheerful or optimistic.

"I was aware that I still had rheumatoid arthritis," she told her friend. "But it just didn't seem important any more. Helping others seemed to overwhelm my awareness of pain."

Wilma also realized that not only had she learned to manage her pain but that she had also gained complete control over it. For as long as she continued to exercise, and to eat healthfully and to stay relaxed, her arthritis pain could never control her life again.

At last report, three years after the doctor first told Wilma she would never walk again without pain, Wilma's arthritis symptoms had gone into remission and she was learning to square dance.

■ THE MAGIC OF BEHAVIORAL MEDICINE

The literature is filled with similar case histories. By being willing to use their minds and muscles, literally millions of Americans have overcome arthritis pain and gone on to lead active and fulfilling lives.

Remember, I'm not claiming to have any magical cure for arthritis. But I do claim that, with your physician's cooperation and approval, you should be able to reduce much of the *pain* of arthritis and to significantly increase the range of motion of arthritic joints.

Arthritis is simply an umbrella term for over 100 different disorders of the joints. The varieties of arthritis range from osteo- and rheumatoid arthritis, the two most common, to gout, allergic reactions that cause inflammatory arthritis, and injuries that result in damage to tendons, bursae, ligaments, muscles, and cartilage. Since therapies that may benefit one type of arthritis could conceivably worsen another type, it is vital to have your arthritis medically diagnosed. A medical diagnosis is also essential to screen out such dangerous forms of arthritis as lupus, polymyalgia rheumatica, or ankylosing spondylitis.

If you wake up stiff and tired, with persistent joint pain, swelling, and tenderness for more than two consecutive weeks or longer you may have arthritis. So arrange to see a doctor as soon as you can. Rheumatoid arthritis pain usually begins in the twenties or thirties, while osteoarthritis seldom appears before age 50. Both varieties are more common in women than in men.

PAINSTOPPER #22:
Speedy Relief for Arthritis Pain

Provided a joint is neither red nor swollen, or hot, applying heat will almost always soothe and release the pain of osteo- or rheumatoid arthritis. By stimulating circulation, heat relaxes the muscles around joints, counteracting stiffness and promoting mobility and flexibility.

One of the best and safest ways to relieve arthritis pain is to take a 20-minute soak in a tub of warm to moderately hot water. Many arthritis sufferers recommend mixing 2 cups of Epsom salts into the bath water or adding bubbles or bath oil. However, it is the hot water that does the trick. Alternatively, you can soak in a hot tub, Jacuzzi®, or whirlpool bath. (Anyone with high blood pressure or a cardiovascular disorder may have to avoid a very hot tub or a whirlpool or Jacuzzi® bath.)

Next best thing is a hot shower. Allow the water to spray on the painful area for several minutes. Then spray the shoulders, neck, and the back, and top of your head for a few minutes. Return and spray the painful area for several more minutes. Then keep alternating. For best results, stay in the shower for 20 minutes or more.

To eliminate early morning stiffness swiftly, take a warm bath or shower as soon as you wake up.

To Ease Pain in a Single Joint

Heat will also soothe and relieve arthritis pain in a single joint. You can apply it with a heating pad, an electric blanket, a hot-water bottle, or a hot pack. Or you can use a heat lamp with an infrared (not ultraviolet) bulb. Place the lamp about 2 feet from the painful joint for 20 – 25 minutes. (To avoid falling asleep and burning yourself, never lie on a heating pad: always apply it over a joint, never underneath.)

For relieving the pain of an acute flare-up of chronic rheumatoid arthritis, moist heat is considered more effective. To apply moist heat, soak a towel in hot water at 116° Fahrenheit, wring out, and place over the afflicted joint. Cover the towel with waxed paper then with a dry towel. You will need to resoak and wring out the towel again every few minutes.

Alternatively, you can make a compress by placing a loaf of bread inside a towel and soaking both in hot water. Remove from the water and twist the towel to wring out the water. Apply the compress to the joint, wrap it in wax paper, and cover with a dry towel. This bread compress will hold heat longer than will a towel alone.

To apply moist heat to fingers, wrists, feet, or ankles, immerse them in a pail of water or in a footbath or small tub. The water should come 6 inches above the ankles, or 6 inches above the wrists, and the temperature should be around 105° F. Immerse hands or feet for 5 full minutes.

Moist heat is a powerful pain reliever, and results are often quite dramatic.

When Cold May Work Better

To relieve arthritis pain, always try heat first. But if heat doesn't work, be prepared to apply cold.

A study made in the 1980s by Peter Utsinger at Germantown Medical Center, Philadelphia, found that direct application of cold to painful joints often succeeded when heat failed. During the study, 240 people with a variety of different forms of arthritis applied ice bags to their afflicted joints once each day. Eighty-five percent experienced a significant decrease in pain and inflammation.

Besides reducing joint temperature, cold inhibits transmission of nerve impulses and also interferes with reception of these impulses in the brain. In the process, cold may also stimulate release of endorphins.

Cold may be particularly helpful in relieving the pain of rheumatoid arthritis in the knees. A four-week trial of 24 rheumatoid arthritis patients with painful knees, also made at Germantown Medical Center, Philadelphia, found that, after four weeks of applying ice, patients reported significant increases in knee range of motion, muscle strength, knee function, and sleep and a decrease in the need for pain-killing drugs. Treatment consisted of placing an ice bag containing six ice cubes and a quart of water above the knee and a similar ice bag below the knee, for 20 minutes 3 times a day. No ill effects occurred, and the results were reported in the *Journal of the American Medical Association,* July 24, 1981.

Similar results might be obtained by using two gel packs and an elastic bandage.

Using Heat and Cold Together

If neither heat by itself nor cold will relieve arthritis pain, then alternate an application of heat with an application of cold. Change over every few minutes. If you use a shower, keep the cold application shorter and avoid running the water so cold that it shocks the body. Keep the spray directed at the painful area.

To apply alternating heat and cold to feet or ankles, or to hands or wrists, you can use pails of hot and cold water. Soak hands or feet in hot water at 105–110° F for several minutes; then immerse them in cold water for the same period of time. Alternate 2 to 3 times until the pain is relieved.

When neither heat nor cold therapy alone works, alternating heat and cold may provide very effective pain relief.

PAINSTOPPER #23:
More Relief for Arthritis Pain

Exercise is the best way to combat the pain and stiffness of osteo- or rheumatoid arthritis. Numerous studies have confirmed that brisk walking, or other forms of exercise, can significantly reduce the extent of arthritis pain.

A study of 102 people with osteoarthritis of the knee (reported in the *Annals of Internal Medicine,* April 1, 1992) found that after participating in a program of walking exercise for eight weeks, the arthritis patients reported feeling considerably less pain, and they used far fewer pain medications, than did a control group that did not exercise. A similar study at Washington University Arthritis Center, St. Louis, confirmed that a vigorous daily walk, or similar exercise, reduced all forms of arthritis pain. In fact, the Arthritis Foundation itself recommends exercise, particularly walking, provided it can be done without discomfort.

In 1986, John H. Bland, a rheumatologist at the University of Vermont, suggested that exercise might even promote the healing of cartilage damaged by osteoarthritis. Bland posited that when a person with arthritis walks, bicycles, or swims for 15 minutes or so, then rests for 1 hour, and keeps repeating this cycle for several hours a day, cartilage in the joints is able to expand more frequently. In this way, cartilage cells might reproduce themselves and eventually repair the damage done by osteoarthritis.

Although Bland's viewpoint is considered controversial, gentle exercise is widely recommended to keep muscles stretched and to increase range of motion. The very worst way to recover from arthritis, or to try and relieve pain, is to lie down all day watching television. Bed rest leads to bone loss and muscle atrophy, both of which worsen arthritis pain and hinder chances for recovery.

This book is based on behavioral medicine, or action therapy. By acting, that is by using our minds and muscles to perform a therapeutic action-step, we *can* offset the ill effects of arthritis and we *can* significantly relieve the pain. This is especially true when we use our muscles to exercise.

For maximum benefit, we need to exercise regularly in two different ways. First, we need to exercise aerobically by walking, bicycling, swimming, or rowing. Second, we need to keep our joints and muscles flexible and mobile by stretching them gently every day.

Warm Up Before You Begin

Everyone with arthritis should try to soak in a tub of warm water for 10 – 15 minutes before exercising. As you warm up in the tub, use slow, gentle movements to free up every joint in the body. Then massage the muscles above and below any arthritic joint.

As you begin to exercise, progress slowly to avoid hurting painful joints and avoid fast, jerky movements. If exercise brings on a muscle tremor, or if pain develops and persists for several hours, you are pushing yourself too hard. After exercising, rest for a period equal to the duration of the exercise. And remember, you will need your doctor's approval before taking up an exercise program.

Aerobic Exercise

Whether you walk, ride a stationary bicycle, swim, or use a rowing machine, brisk, rhythmic exercise benefits every cell in the body. Never push yourself too hard. But try, if you can, eventually to work up to where your pulse and respiratory rates are elevated as you exercise for 35 minutes or more. At this point, your brain will begin to release endorphin, the body's natural morphine pain-killer. Endorphins bind with pain receptors in the brain, significantly decreasing the experience of pain for the remainder of the day.

- *Walking.* Anyone with arthritis absolutely must wear a well-cushioned pair of athletic fitness walking shoes for aerobic walking. Don't even think about walking in cheap discount store jogging shoes or in high-heeled shoes or in shoes with thin soles. Many people with arthritis walk daily in malls throughout the year. Begin by walking for 20 minutes if you can, then gradually increase distance and speed.

- *Bicycling.* A zero-impact exercise, bicycling is especially recommended for people with arthritis of the hips or knees. On a stationary bicycle, set the resistance to "low" to begin with and increase gradually. To adjust seat height correctly, the leg should be almost, but not quite, straight when the pedal reaches its lowest point.

- *Rowing Machines.* Rowing is recommended for building upper body strength and mobility as well as for aerobic benefit. Begin with 10 minutes a day and increase gradually to 20 minutes or more.

- *Swimming.* This is another impact-free exercise that stresses only the shoulders. If you're unable to swim, walk along the bottom of the pool while standing waist deep in water and use the hands as paddles to help you along.

Avoid any exercise that involves deep knee bends, contact sports, or heavy weight lifting. And always stop if you feel any pain.

■ INCREASING YOUR STRENGTH HELPS OVERCOME ARTHRITIS PAIN

For anyone with osteoarthritis of the knee, good muscle tone is essential to keep the joint functioning. A short workout every other day on a Nautilus-type leg extender machine is the best way to build up the quadricep muscles in the thigh. The same machine also lets you build up the opposing hamstring muscles.

If you do not have access to a Nautilus-type machine (found in virtually all health spas and gyms), you can strengthen your quadriceps like this. Sit in an upright chair with both feet flat on the floor. Straighten the knee so that one leg is stretched out in front. Lower it back down again. Next, place a light weight on your foot, such as a small bag of sand, and raise your leg up and down as many times as you can. Repeat with the other knee. Place enough weight on your foot to offer some resistance. Gradually increase the weight as your quadriceps become stronger. As you get into heavier weights, you may want to sit on the floor with knees flexed and support the exercising knee with a pile of cushions.

Working out with light to moderate weights is another excellent way for anyone with arthritis to build strength. Interestingly, studies at both Tufts and Harvard universities have confirmed that 90-year-old people with arthritis have improved their ability to walk after working out with weights 3 times a week.

Use moderate weights at first until you can do 13 repetitions of an exercise. Then increase the weight to the next step and do as many reps as you can.

■ STRETCHING BENEFITS ALL TYPES OF ARTHRITIS

Exercises that stretch the joints and muscles reduce contraction of joints and shortening of muscles and muscle spasm. When stretching is combined with aerobic exercise, mobility and range of motion are increased, fatigue is reduced, and posture is improved. Stretching is particularly beneficial during a flare-up of rheumatoid arthritis, and it helps to reduce all types of pain.

For maximum benefit, you should stretch for 15 minutes a day 5 or . more times a week. Here are some stretching exercises specifically designed to help people with arthritis.

Chin Tuck and Stretch

Remain seated in a chair throughout the seven steps of this exercise.

- *Step 1:* Keeping your head level, like a Thai dancer, pull your chin back as though making a double chin. Then slide the head all the way forward so that the chin sticks out. Repeat 10 times.

- *Step 2:* Tilt the head up and back as far as you can. Then gently lower the chin to the chest and drop your head as low as you can. Repeat several times.

- *Step 3:* Slowly tilt and stretch the head all the way to the left, trying to touch your left shoulder with your left ear. Then stretch the head in the opposite direction. Repeat 5 times each way.

- *Step 4:* Slowly rotate the head as far as you can to the left, then as far as you can to the right.

- *Step 5:* Relax the neck and head and slowly do a neck roll. That is, roll the head down on your chest, then over to the right, then far back, then to the left, and finally down to the front again. Repeat 3 times in each direction.

- *Step 6:* Open your mouth as wide as possible and stick out your tongue as far as you can. Hold for 10 seconds, or longer, and release.

- *Step 7:* Raise one shoulder at a time as far as you can, then lower it. Raise and lower the other shoulder. Repeat 5 times with each shoulder. As you become more limber, rotate the shoulder in a circular direction as well as up and down. Then rotate it in the opposite direction.

Elbow Stretch

Sit on a chair. Keeping the arms straight, clasp the hands together in front of you. Bend the elbows and bring your clasped hands up to your left shoulder. Then, as you straighten the elbows, lower your hands to your right knee. Next, bring your hands to your right shoulder and left knee. Alternate for 20 repetitions.

Finger Stretch

Sit on a chair. Close your fists and hold for 5 seconds. Open your hands as wide as possible. Keep your fingers straight and bend back your wrists. Hold for 5 seconds. Repeat the entire exercise 20 times.

As you progress, bend the wrists down as you make a fist and bend them all the way back as you open your hands.

Shoulder Stretch

Stand with your legs a moderate distance apart and hold onto the back of a chair with one hand. Bend forward from the waist. Let your other free arm hang loose, with your hand dangling near the floor. Gently, begin to trace small circles with your hand. As your arm limbers up, make the circles larger. Repeat with the other hand.

Upper Back Stretch

Lie on your back on the floor on a rug or carpet. Place your arms at your sides, hands with palms down. Flex your knees and keep your feet flat on the floor. Cross the right leg over the left leg. Then twist your torso all the way to the right, turning your shoulders as far around as you can and turning your head to look over your right shoulder.

Repeat on the other side. Then repeat 4 more times in each direction. As you become more limber, try the same exercise while sitting up on the floor.

The Cobra Stretch

Lie face down on the floor on a comfortable rug or carpet. Place your hands on the rug, palms down, under your shoulders. Gently raise the shoulders a few inches off the floor, causing your spine to arch. Hold for 5 seconds and lower.

Repeat up to 5 times. As your spine becomes more flexible, you will be able to go higher. As you do, raise your head as high as you can and hold it there. You will then be in the classic yoga posture known as the cobra pose.

Trunk Twist

Lie on your back on a floor rug or carpet with your knees flexed and feet flat on the floor. Slowly twist the hips to the left as far as you can until your knees touch the floor. Meanwhile, keep your shoulders flat on the floor. Hold 5 seconds and return to the starting postition. Twist in the same way to the right. Repeat several times in each direction.

Side Stretch

Sit upright in a chair with feet about twelve inches apart and knees uncrossed. Bend your trunk down to the left and touch the floor with your left fingers. Straighten up and repeat to the right. Repeat 5 times each way.

Achilles Stretch

Place a thick book, or a short length of 2-inch × 4-inch lumber, flat on the floor so that it forms a step about 2 inches high. Hold on to a wall, doorpost, or chair; then place the balls of both feet on the step. Gently raise up on the toes as high as you can; then lower your heels down to the floor. Repeat up to 10 times. As you gain strength and flexibility, add another book to raise the step another inch. Eventually, do the exercise with only one foot at a time.

OSTEOARTHRITIS

■ WHAT YOU SHOULD KNOW ABOUT OSTEOARTHRITIS

A key step in overcoming any type of pain by natural means is to first learn all you can about it. Knowing how a pain occurs and what causes it gives you a tremendous sense of power over that pain. This is especially true with arthritis.

The following story was told to me by the husband of Joan R., a Midwestern housewife, who became crippled with osteoarthritis (O-A).

Several years ago, he said, his wife had become addicted to watching television, and much of her day was spent lying down watching the screen and munching junk food. Within months, her weight had ballooned to 200 pounds, and she began to wake up with stiffness in her knees and spine. Whenever she walked, her knees and upper back would ache, and only rest would relieve the pain.

Her doctor diagnosed osteoarthritis and he prescribed a series of expensive nonsteroid anti-inflammatory drugs. They relieved some of the pain, but Joan's condition continued to deteriorate. Tiny pieces of cartilage would break off in her knees and cause redness and swelling and even more pain. Meanwhile, the bone ends in Joan's knees began to break down. Her body responded with an overgrowth of new bone in the form of painful spurs. These spurs made Joan's knees look deformed. One of her knees became unstable and began to wobble.

Joan remained completely unaware that there was anything she could do for her O-A except to take pain pills. One evening, she watched a television program on arthritis. The narrator said that being overweight and sedentary was the underlying cause of most O-A. He said that, by doing exactly the opposite—by losing weight and exercising—the pain could be lessened and further damage halted.

A rheumatologist (arthritis specialist) then confirmed that, although worn cartilage could not be replaced, anyone willing to lose weight and exercise might reasonably expect to rehabilitate an afflicted joint.

The TV program gave Joan a glimmer of hope.

"I hated being fat and housebound," she said. "For the first time in years I began to suspect that I could do something to improve my condition."

Becoming a Medically Informed Layperson Gives Joan R. New Hope

Joan began driving to the library and spending her days reading everything she could find about O-A. In less than a week, she had gathered a wealth of information. As the TV program had predicted, her O-A was due to overloading her weight-bearing joints with excess weight caused by overeating on a high-fat diet. Failing to exercise caused her weight to soar even more. And lack of movement made her joints so stiff that they had already lost most of their range of motion.

As Joan learned, while excessive use of a joint, or an injury, *can* damage joint cartilage, the most common cause of O-A is being overweight and ignoring the need for exercise. Most of the 16 million Americans who have O-A are either heavyweight women who eat unwisely and rarely exercise, or heavy muscular men who lead sedentary lives. Joan read that many of the men are former athletes or football players who are no longer active. She also learned that O-A is seldom seen in athletes who have stayed trim and fit. In fact, arthritis of any sort is rare in vegetarian men and women who remain fit and active.

As the days went by, Joan became increasingly aware that obesity imposes a serious overload on weight-bearing cartilage in the knees, hips, neck, and spine—the principal joints where O-A strikes. Women are also frequently afflicted with O-A in the fingers where it causes hard, bony nodules and neuritis pain. But actual damage to these nonweight-bearing joints is seldom enough to impair movement.

Medical Know-how Helps Joan R. Develop a Strategy to Beat Arthritis Pain

As was true in Joan's case, O-A appears most often in women in the knees and upper spine. Spinal O-A in women may lead to stiffness in the neck, arms, and shoulders or may even cause headache, earache, or sore throat.

In men, O-A most commonly strikes in the hips and lower spine. Hip pain often spreads to the groin and to inside the thigh. O-A in the base of the spine may also spread across the lower back. Joan recalled a male friend with O-A in the base of the spine. The man was scared to death of coughing or sneezing because to do so would trigger a severe stabbing pain in the lower spine.

Joan also recognized herself when she read that, since O-A pain is worsened by movement, most victims tend to avoid moving around. Stiffness then becomes chronic, and soon, the sufferer adopts the familiar arthritis shuffle or limp.

Also contributing to O-A is the standard American diet that is low in fiber and high in fat. Such diets are almost always lacking in fruits, vegetables, whole grains, and legumes and are often deficient in calcium and magnesium. In a sedentary, overweight person, lack of calcium and magnesium can lead to osteoporosis or weakening of the skeletal bones.

Joan felt concerned when she realized that she herself was a prime candidate for osteoporosis and a possible broken hip.

Joan quickly discovered that she could relieve her pain with heat and movement (our Painstoppers #22 and #23). But these techniques would relieve her discomfort only until bedtime. Next day, she had to repeat them over again.

Putting together all she had learned, Joan roughed out a game plan designed to bring more permanent and lasting relief from O-A pain. Her strategy is described next.

PAINSTOPPER #24:
The Ultimate Way to Reduce Osteoarthritis Pain

To achieve lasting relief from O-A pain, Joan recognized that she must be willing to step outside her comfort zone and make several key life-style changes. For starters, she and her husband agreed to watch only one hour of television each day. The rest of the time, the set stayed switched off. Her game plan then looked like this.

MY GOAL: To reduce weight down to normal (140 pounds) for my height and build. I will achieve this through steps 1 and 2.

- *Step 1:* I will change to a heart-healthy diet. I will adopt immediately a high-fiber, plant-based diet in which less than 15 percent of calories is derived from fat. I will reduce by 75 percent all flesh foods, eggs, dairy foods, fats, and oils and anything containing white flour or sugar. At the same time, I will quadruple my intake of fruits, vegetables, legumes, and whole grains. I will also eliminate all fried foods.

  I will begin each day with a hearty breakfast of whole-grain cereals and four helpings of fruit. Lunch will be a large, raw vegetable salad. And dinner will be a slightly smaller meal of steamed vegetables and whole grains. For snacks I will eat only plain, air-popped popcorn, fruits, carrots, celery, pretzels, or whole wheat fig bars.

  Joan's diet was virtually identical to that in our Painstopper #3: The One Diet That Does It All. Look up this painstopper in Chapter 3 for complete details.

- *Step 2:* I will steadily increase my level of physical exertion. As I lose fat, which lowers my metabolism, I will build up muscle, which increases my metabolism. The higher my metabolism, the faster I will burn off fat and keep it off. Since my arms, hips, and abdomen are unaffected by arthritis, I will start using strength-building exercises to restore muscle in these areas.

  As I steadily lose weight through exercise and sound nutrition, it will lower the weight-bearing stress on my spine and knees. As my weight falls, I shall begin bicycling and, later, walking.

  Once I am able to walk again, I will gradually work into a daily aerobic walking program. (At this point, Joan's program would be identical to that of our Painstopper #2: Walk Away from Pain, described in Chapter 3.)

- *Step 3:* I will question my doctor's choice of medication. I believe my doctor is prescribing pain medication on the basis of drug company advertising. As soon as possible, I plan to ask him to replace these expensive anti-inflammatory drugs with two 325-mg plain aspirin to be taken four times each day. Or if I can't take aspirin, then I'll use acetaminophen or ibuprofen.

  I also plan to take 1 gram of supplemental calcium daily and 400 mg of magnesium to help my bones rebuild and to prevent osteoporosis.

Scientific Proof That Osteoarthritis Pain Can Be Reduced Without Drugs

It took self-discipline and motivation to carry out these action-steps. But whenever she found herself vacillating, Joan would use stop-go switching to get back on track (see our Painstopper #6: Stop Pain-Provoking Habits with a Rubber Band).

Whenever Joan felt like going on a binge, she would remind herself of a study done at Boston University School of Medicine. Based on a survey of 64 women with recently diagnosed O-A of the knee and 728 women without this condition, researchers developed a model which showed that a woman 5 feet 11 inches in height who lost 11 pounds in weight over a 10 year period, could cut her risk of developing O-A by 50 percent. Women with shorter or heavier builds can achieve this same degree of protection by losing weight roughly in proportion to that of the tall woman in the sample.

This means that provided your weight does not fall below the optimal level for your height and build, the more weight you lose, the more you reduce the risk of ever getting O-A of the knee.

The study's authors concluded that even if you already have O-A of the knee and are overweight, shedding excess weight can still help relieve pain and minimize further damage.

"I'm not easily impressed by anecdotal case histories," Joan told her husband. "But here is actual scientific proof that losing weight can help relieve osteoarthritis pain in weight-bearing joints. I've read that 10 percent of people aged 65 and over have osteoarthritis of the knee. They're nearly all women, and they're nearly all overweight. They continue to have pain because they refuse to lose weight."

Joan was determined to succeed. To ensure that she lost 1 pound per week, she weighed herself every morning on awakening and again before dinner. Each week, her weight had to be one pound less than the previous week. If it wasn't, she cut her next meal in half, and she continued to eat only half as much as normal until her weight *did* drop by 1 pound. Using this simple method, she found she could usually control her weight loss by reducing the size of her final meal of the day.

Joan R. Beats the Agony of Osteoarthritis

No, Joan didn't lose her osteoarthritis. But just over a year later, when her weight had dropped to 140 pounds, she found she could walk half a mile at a time with almost no pain. Her stiffness had disappeared entirely, and she had become so flexible that she had enrolled in a yoga class. She no longer needed aspirin or any pain-killing drugs. And she had virtually eliminated all foods of animal origin, including eggs and dairy foods, from her diet.

"There's no magic food that will stop the pain of osteoarthritis," she tells her friends. "But diet was still the key to relieving my arthritis pain. My osteoarthritis was entirely due to the impact of 60 surplus pounds crushing the cartilage in my knees and spine at every step."

"The brief pleasure of eating fatty foods wasn't worth all that pain," she continues. "Today, I get just as much taste pleasure from eating different, healthier foods. If you have osteoarthritis pain in a weight-bearing joint, you can lessen your pain and may get rid of it entirely, by cutting your weight back down to normal."

RHEUMATOID ARTHRITIS

■ WHAT YOU SHOULD KNOW ABOUT RHEUMATOID ARTHRITIS

Rheumatoid arthritis (R-A) is a progressive, systematic disease that may not only destroy cartilage and cause inflammation in joints, but may also involve muscles, tendons, ligaments, and even bones, heart, lungs, eyes, mouth, and blood vessels.

As this was written, many researchers agreed that R-A appears to be caused by our immune system's response to a superantigen triggered by a virus or bacteria. The immune system produces billions of specialized killer T-cells to destroy the superantigen. But the superantigen is able to ward off this massive attack. Meanwhile, the hordes of killer T-cells, roving the body in search of *something* to attack and destroy, turn on the body's own cartilage and begin to destroy healthy cells. In the process, they cause inflammation and pain and stiffness in joints, accompanied by varying degrees of muscle ache, overwhelming fatigue and weakness, anemia, loss of weight and appetite, and general malaise.

This aberration of the immune system can spread throughout the body. It may cause extensive and irreparable damage to joints. Fingers and toes may become grotesquely distorted, twisted, and useless. Ankles, knees, wrists, hips, shoulders, and elbows are other common targets, and frequently the same joint is afflicted on both sides of the body.

R-A strikes three times as many women as men — frequently between ages 20 and 45 — and especially during the stress of child rearing. Curiously, once a woman with R-A becomes pregnant, she obtains immediate relief from the disease — often for good. In men, R-A often strikes in the spinal area.

How Rheumatologists Classify Rheumatoid Arthritis Pain

Rheumatologists classify R-A on a scale of 1 to 4. Class 1 is the mildest, Class 4 the most severe. In people with Class 1 or 2, the disease may smoulder much of the time and surface periodically with a brief flare-up of symptoms. People with Class 3 or 4 experience more severe symptoms, characterized by hot, swollen, and painful joints and, often, a low-grade fever. Forty percent of people with Class 3 or 4 R-A find it difficult to walk, sew, climb stairs, or open doors, and some experience emotional depression. Nonetheless, most people with R-A are able to function fairly well, and only a small number are permanently or severely crippled.

The nature of R-A with its periodic flare-ups that then subside, often for months, makes it difficult to identify a true remission. However, over time, pain tends to decrease and R-A burns itself out and disappears.

In 1987, Dr. Lewis Kazis, assistant research professor of medicine at Boston University Medical Center, made a study of 261 people who had had R-A for an average of nine years. The group was tested for disabilities and then given the same test five years later. Dr. Kazis found no significant decrease in their level of physical activity, manual dexterity, or ability to carry out daily activities. On a long-term basis, Dr. Kazis concluded that the health status of people with R-A remains remarkably stable.

While a small number of R-A victims do experience a decline in health, the majority appear not to deteriorate either physically or mentally. This was confirmed by another Massachusetts study of 118 people who displayed symptoms of R-A. When these same 118 people were examined three to five years later, fewer than one in three still displayed R-A symptoms. The study authors concluded that 25 percent of people with R-A should permanently recover within three to five years, 50 percent will have mild to moderate symptoms, and only 25 percent will be classified as Class 3 or 4.

Medical Treatment for Severe Rheumatoid Arthritis is Vigorous and Aggressive

Obviously, if you have any symptoms of R-A, you should see your doctor or a rheumatologist without delay. Yet the real risk lies in having R-A of Class 4 severity. The disease may do extensive damage during the first few years, permanently crippling and disabling joints, seriously affecting a person's quality of life, and even threatening life itself.

Nowadays, the main thrust of medical treatment is to vigorously and aggressively treat Class 4 R-A to halt the progress of the disease and to stop inflammation and joint destruction before serious damage can occur.

To achieve this goal, a powerful combination of gold salts, steroids, and immunosuppressive drugs is frequently prescribed. Unfortunately, many people find the drugs' side effects as bad, or worse, than the symptoms of R-A. Considering the serious nature of Class 4 R-A, the treatment undoubtedly makes sense. But side effects of these drugs—they're called disease-modifying anti rheumatic drugs (often abbreviated as DMARDs)—range from skin rash to mouth ulcers to osteoporosis, immunosuppression (which increases the risk of cancer and infections), reduced vision, nausea, and possible liver damage, or lung and kidney problems. The drugs are very slow acting and must be taken over a long period of time. And since it will take some 20 years to assess their effectiveness, the vigorous treatment of severe R-A with DMARDs is still considered a new and experimental approach. As symptoms gradually subside, milder drugs are substituted. But this could take several years.

PAINSTOPPER #25:
A Scientifically Proven All-Natural Way to Alleviate the Pain and Inflammation of Rheumatoid Arthritis

We may not be able to cure or prevent R-A by diet, but a variety of recent studies indicate that, for many people, diet may help to alleviate the pain, inflammation, and stiffness caused by R-A.

The gist of the studies is that the inflammation in R-A is intensified by the prostaglandin leukotriene, a hormonelike substance produced from omega-6 type fatty acids found in many vegetable oils and in foods of animal origin. Fish oil, by comparison, contains omega-3 fatty acids, which the body does not transform into the type of leukotriene that causes inflammation.

During the studies it was also found that olive and canola oils play a neutral role in contributing to inflammation. Although participants in the studies took fish oil supplements, it has since been found that eating fish three to five or more times a week is more effective and more palatable. Cod liver oil should never be taken.

Instead, many nutritionists now recommend eating an oily fish such as tuna, halibut, mackerel, sardines packed in water (not in vegetable oil), or salmon.

In one study at Boston's Brigham and Women's Hospital, 33 people with Class 1, 2, or 3 R-A reported at least 30 minutes of morning stiffness with tender and swollen joints. For 14 weeks, half the group then took fish oil supplements and the other half took a placebo. The two groups then switched places. In both cases, those taking fish oil reported an average decrease of one-third in joint tenderness, and they were free of fatigue for $2\frac{1}{2}$ hours longer each day. Almost identical results were reported during similar studies at Albany Medical College and at Harvard Medical School and the Royal Adelaide Hospital, Australia. Study results were documented in several leading medical journals.

From The Netherlands comes word of yet other studies in which participants significantly reduced the pain, stiffness, and inflammation of R-A by eschewing all foods of animal origin and adopting an exclusively plant-based diet. While becoming a vegetarian may not work for every R-A victim, these findings make sense because they concur with recommendations by virtually all leading health advisory agencies that we can significantly reduce risk of heart disease, cancer, diabetes, and other killer diseases by reducing the fat and oil in our diets and the amount of animal protein.

Based on these findings, it would seem prudent to cut out all fried foods and all fats and oils except small amounts of olive or canola oil. We should also eliminate all whole-milk dairy products, margarine, eggs, and all but nonfat salad dressings. We should then replace as much of the meat and poultry in our diet as possible with three to five or more servings of oily fish each week.

Better still, adopt an exclusively plant-based diet. Some European researchers have speculated that a diet high in flesh foods, fats, and oils gradually blocks arteries with cholesterol plaque. This reduces the supply of oxygen and other nutrients to cartilage and cells in joint areas. Lack of oxygen then helps to speed cartilage breakdown.

Based on the studies, it may take 3 to 6 months for noticeable pain relief to appear. At the same time, however, you will be steadily reducing your risk of ever getting heart disease, cancer, diabetes, and other degenerative diseases.

To get started, look up Painstopper #3: The One Diet That Does It All (in Chapter 3) and follow its guidelines.

PAINSTOPPER #26:
How Sleeping Warm May Eliminate Morning Pain and Stiffness

Staying warm and snug all night is a proven way to prevent the morning pain, stiffness, and swelling associated with R-A.

In 1987, for instance, a study by Peggy McKnight, former director of St. Margaret's Memorial Hospital, Pittsburgh, tested 30 R-A victims who complained of morning pain and stiffness in wrists and hands. The participants were instructed to wear unlined stretch gloves — widely available in drug, department, or medical stores — during sleep. Besides being warm, these gloves exert pressure on hands and wrists. After sleeping in the gloves for seven nights, 21 patients reported less pain, 24 reported less stiffness, and 27 experienced less swelling.

If your morning stiffness is in the knee or elbow, consider cutting a thick knee sock into a tube about 10 inches long and placing it over the afflicted joint. Alternatively, you can wrap a cotton, or a wool scarf, around the joint and keep it in place with an elastic bandage.

Even better results have been reported by R-A victims who sleep in a warm sleeping bag. A sleeping bag (placed on your bed) keeps the body uniformly warm and snug all over. Although more expensive, it is considered far superior to an electric blanket. In recent surveys, hundreds of people who sleep in goosedown bags report having eliminated morning stiffness almost completely.

If you prefer to use regular blankets and comforters on your bed, you can probably avoid waking up stiff and painful by switching on an electric blanket for half an hour before rising.

PAINSTOPPER #27:
Ending Skin Hemorrhaging Due to Rheumatoid Arthritis

Many women with R-A, and some men, are bothered by spontaneous bruising, which causes skin fragility and hemorrhaging. In a small study at Haywood Hospital, Stoke-on-Trent, England, doctors found that administering 500 mg of vitamin C orally each day to women with R-A ended most problems of bruising and hemorrhaging. The explanation appears to be that an ample supply of vitamin C decreases capillary fragility, thus preventing hemorrhage. The healing power of the vitamin C appears to be increased when bioflavinoid supplements are also taken. Many nutritionists believe that R-A depletes the body of vitamin C, while many drugs used to treat R-A inhibit vitamin C metabolism.

PAINSTOPPER #28:
How to Sleep Soundly With Rheumatoid Arthritis

Fatigue and sleeplessness intensify the pain of R-A. Especially during a flare-up, try to sleep at least 8–9 hours each night.

To minimize pain while sleeping, lie on your back with all joints straight. Try to avoid bending or curling the arms, wrists, fingers, elbows, hips, knees, or toes. Keep them relaxed, not rigid, but try to avoid bending any joints during the acute stage of an R-A flare-up. Keep your palms turned up.

You can help keep the knees straight by placing towels under the ankles. However, avoid placing pillows under the knees since it causes unnecessary bending of knee joints. For added comfort, place a folded towel under each wrist and arm to help keep them straight.

Avoid sleeping on your stomach. If you must change your sleeping position, turn on to your side with knees drawn up. Most arthritis sufferers sleep best on a fairly firm mattress. You can probably firm up your mattress by placing a ¾-inch plywood board beneath it.

During R-A flare-ups, try to take at least one brief break during the day. If you can, lie down in a quiet room with the lights off for at least 20 minutes once each day. Actually, a 2-hour nap may be the best immediate solution to R-A pain. However, extended bed rest can be harmful. See Painstopper #23 for gentle movements that you can alternate with rest.

Whenever you're up and about, try to maintain an erect posture and sit only on upright chairs.

PAINSTOPPER #29:
Eliminating the Stress That May Trigger Rheumatoid Arthritis Pain

Many rheumatologists believe that R-A has a strong emotional component and the R-A flare-ups appear after an emotional upset or a period of severe emotional stress. It is believed that fear-based negative emotions in the mind are communicated by neuropeptide messengers to the immune system, triggering the immunoaberrations that precipitate R-A. It has also been pointed out that many R-A victims are people with a high level of emotional and psychological stress. For many years, doctors have also noticed that people with R-A are often pessimistic and have a resentful outlook.

There is no doubt that muscular tension caused by stress can also worsen arthritis pain. All evidence points to the fact that if you can prevent emotional stress or upset, the painful flare-ups of R-A may never occur.

To prevent negative emotions from causing R-A flare-ups, I recommend that you study and adopt the following painstopper action steps.

Painstopper #7: Learning to Beat Pain with Abdominal Breathing
Painstopper #9: Relaxation Training—Nature's Prescription for Pain Relief
Painstopper #11: Biofeedback Training—Mind Over Pain
Painstopper #21: Keep Pain at Bay with Positive Beliefs

I also recommend reading and adopting all the action-steps in Chapter 7, Drive Out Pain with Positive Beliefs, including the Ten Affirmations That May Help Reduce Stress and Relieve Your Chronic Pain.

Many people with R-A have also noticed a decrease in pain through becoming more assertive and by refusing to allow themselves to be used as doormats by others. Burying or repressing negative emotions appears to release hormones that often trigger a flare-up. If this sounds like you, consider the benefits of becoming more assertive and refusing to let other people walk all over you.

Some physicians have also noted that R-A often begins after a severe cold or infection has overloaded the immune system. Whenever another cold or infection occurs, a painful flare-up often follows.

The solution is to lead a healthy life-style based on a balanced mix of sleep, relaxation, and exercise so that you minimize risk of acquiring a cold or infection. If, instead, you lead a helter-skelter life-style filled with physical and emotional stress, you may have identified the cause of your R-A pain.

GOUT

■ WHAT YOU SHOULD KNOW ABOUT GOUT

Fred R. loved rich foods and wines. By his 40th birthday, Fred had developed a portly, middle-aged spread, and the thought of exercising never crossed his mind.

A few weeks later, Fred woke up in the middle of the night with a terrible, searing, throbbing pain in his right big toe. The skin around his toe was red and swollen and hot to the touch while the toe itself was exquisitely tender.

A few days later, after a lab test, Fred's doctor confirmed the pain as due to gout (also called gouty arthritis or crystal arthritis). The physician explained that most cases of gout appear in men over the age of 35. Gout is brought on by unhealthy living habits centered on a diet high in fats, and rich foods and meats, that contain excessive levels of purines.

Once in the body, purines break down to produce an abnormally high concentration of uric acid. This surplus uric acid then combines with other minerals to form urates, or needlelike crystals, that are deposited in and around joints in the feet, wrists, elbows, or knees.

Any movement in these joints then becomes excruciatingly painful. In the early stages, gout attacks seldom last more than ten days.

"But if you continue to indulge in rich foods, and in other unhealthful habits, attacks will become more frequent and the pain will become more severe," the doctor told Fred.

The physician also explained that gout can easily be eliminated by behavioral medicine, in this case by acting to change the life-style behaviors that are causing the gout.

"But most men are unwilling to make the changes," the doctor said. "So we try to treat gout with drugs. The drugs actually do nothing but mask symptoms. And as any gout patient can tell you, most gout medication has very unpleasant side effects."

"It's easier to remove the cause of gout than to try and treat the pain," the doctor continued. "Which do you prefer: to get rid of gout altogether or to palliate it with unpleasant and expensive medication so that you can continue to indulge in a health-wrecking life-style?"

"Sounds like a choice between life or death," Fred said.

"It very well might be," the doctor replied. "If you keep up your present diet and way of life, your gout pain is likely to spread into other joints, and you may well end up with kidney stones and kidney disease."

Fred paused and reflected briefly.

"All that indulgent eating and rich living wasn't really much fun," he admitted. "The heck with making the drug companies rich. I really needed a shock like this to jolt me out of it. I'll do anything to never have this pain again. Tell me what I have to do."

The advice the doctor gave Fred is summarized in Painstopper #30.

PAINSTOPPER #30:
The Ultimate Way to End the Pain of Gout Forever

With very few exceptions, the pain of gout can be ended, once and for all, by adopting and practicing the six action-steps that follow. The only possible exception may be a few cases of people who have a genetic predisposition to gout. And they, also, would be likely to benefit by making these action-steps an integral part of their life-style.

As always, before using any natural technique for reducing pain, you should have your gout medically diagnosed, and you should have your doctor's approval before using any of these action-steps.

- *Step 1:* Eliminate alcohol entirely. Use Painstoppers #5 and #6 to help cut your alcohol consumption by one drink per day until it reaches zero.

- *Step 2:* Eliminate all purines from the diet. Foods high in purines include all organ meats, such as liver, kidney, brains, heart and sweetbreads; goose or duck meat and pate de foie gras; anchovies, asparagus, bouillon, condiments, consomme, gravies, herring, meat extracts, mincemeat, mushrooms, mussels, sardines, smoked fish, and most rich or fatty meats and seafood. In fact, almost any kind of fat, oil, meat, poultry, or seafood is likely to contain uric acid–forming purines. Beverages containing caffeine, such as coffee, tea, cocoa, and chocolate, also contain xanthines, another precursor of uric acid.

  To make a clean sweep of all harmful nutrients, I recommend adopting and following Painstopper #3: The One Diet That Does It All. In the process, you will not only rid yourself of gout but also dramatically lower your risk of ever getting such painful conditions as heart disease or cancer.

- *Step 3:* Lower body weight to normal. Again, I recommend achieving this step by adopting Painstopper #3, which will lower your weight gradually and without dieting. At all costs, avoid any crash diet or low-calorie diet or fasting. Each of these techniques may cause a drastic increase in uric acid level and lead to a flare-up of gout. Weight loss must be gradual and spread out over a period of weeks or months.

For anyone with gout, the best way to lose weight is to steadily reduce dietary fat and animal protein while simultaneously increasing intake of complex carbohydrates (fruits, vegetables, legumes, and whole grains).

- *Step 4:* Increase fluid intake. Drink much, much more nonalcoholic fluids. To prevent kidney stones from forming, to help complex carbohydrate digestion, and to help uric acid crystals to gradually dissolve, drink at least 3 quarts of fluid daily.

- *Step 5:* Begin a program of gradually increasing daily exercise. I recommend using Painstopper #2: Walk Away from Pain to achieve this step.

- *Step 6:* Replace nutrients that are frequently depleted by gout. People with gout are often deficient in vitamins B, C, and E. To restore these nutrient levels, several nutritionists have advised taking 1 gram of supplemental vitamin C daily together with vitamin E, and a B-complex supplement containing folic acid. All are freely available in health food stores. You should not exceed the manufacturer's recommended daily dosages. Taking megadoses of vitamins, especially of vitamin C or niacin, may hinder rather than help recovery from gout.

Fred lost no time in following all six of his doctor's recommendations. His gout didn't disappear immediately. He suffered two more painful flare-ups. But Fred firmly believed that he would shake off his gout, and he persisted and stayed with his program. This strong belief helped his placebo power and enabling effect to kick in. For the first time in years, Fred began to actually enjoy being alive.

In the three years that have elapsed since his last gout attack, Fred's health has improved enormously. He is 40 pounds lighter, he looks at least 10 years younger, and he has become an avid walker and tennis player.

PAINSTOPPER #31:
A Tasty Fruit That May Reduce the Pain of Gout

One man who faithfully followed all six action steps in Painstopper #30 still occasionally suffered from a flare-up of gout. The reason, his doctor discovered, was that he had a genetic predisposition to gout.

This man discovered that by eating half a pound of cherries each day, he could eliminate any further flare-ups of gout. He kept a can of pie cherries in his refrigerator and he ate 2 ounces of cherries four times each day. As long as he did, his gout remained in remission. But if he stopped eating the cherries, the gout would eventually flare up once more.

Call it folklore, or an example of the placebo effect at work, but many former gout victims have also claimed that eating cherries has helped them end the pain of gout more swiftly. In general, the advice is to eat half a pound of red or black cherries, preferably fresh, or else in canned or frozen form. Equally beneficial results have been reported by eating blueberries or hawthorne berries. If the berries themselves are not available, most health food stores carry extracts of these berries. Adding watercress or parsley to salads or other foods also seems to have helped some people.

One explanation is that all these foods are rich sources of flavenoids, a nutrient that lowers uric acid levels and, as a result, may reduce the pain of gout in joints. Additionally, cherries and similar fruits are complex carbohydrates. And the more complex carbohydrates you put in your stomach, the less room there is for foods containing purines.

Certainly, this nutritional tip sounds worth trying, especially if you enjoy eating cherries. Consider mixing the cherries with other fruits to form a tasty fruit salad topped with plain, nonfat yogurt. You may have to eat cherries for several weeks before results appear.

BURSITIS AND TENDINITIS

■ WHAT YOU SHOULD KNOW ABOUT BURSITIS

The body has over 140 bursae or fluid-filled sacs that cushion muscles as they glide across large joints. When, due to an injury, or to overuse, a bursa is damaged and dries out, it no longer provides a cushioning effect. Instead, the bursa swells up and becomes inflamed. Thereafter, the slightest movement becomes exquisitely painful.

Since bursitis frequently results from overuse by such repetitive movements as scrubbing, sandpapering, or sawing, it strikes most often in the shoulder, elbow, knee, hip, foot, or groin. The acutely painful period usually lasts for 4 to 7 days, after which the pain gradually subsides. Generally, all pain is gone by the 14th day.

For either bursitis or tendinitis immediate first aid should consist of RICE, that is, rest, ice, compression, and elevation. Cut back on activity, apply an icepack to the injured area, compress the injured area by wrapping it in an elastic bandage, and keep the area elevated.

Should the acute stage of pain not subside within a week, or if redness, heat, or fever appear, you should see a doctor. The joint may be infected. Both bursitis and tendinitis are often misdiagnosed or are confused with referred pain from spinal arthritis or a pinched spinal nerve. Even if correctly diagnosed, there often isn't much that a doctor can do for either bursitis or tendinitis.

A well-placed injection of cortisone or xylocaine may relieve persistent bursitis pain. But doctors often miss the target area, resulting in distinctly uncomfortable side effects. Surgery may be used as a last resort for chronic bursitis.

Fortunately, the outlook for natural healing is far more optimistic. The action-steps that follow should end the pain of bursitis or tendinitis in the shortest possible time.

■ WHAT YOU SHOULD KNOW ABOUT TENDINITIS

A tendon is a band of tissue that attaches muscle fiber to bone. When a tendon becomes inflamed, the pain is called *tendinitis*. Tendinitis can be caused by any sudden physical or mechanical stress such as a sudden stop while exercising or while making an improper backhand stroke in tennis. Tendinitis occurs most often in the elbow, shoulder, hip, or foot. Bursitis and tendinitis often occur together, particularly in the shoulder.

PAINSTOPPER #32:
How to End Bursitis Pain

Perhaps the swiftest way to end bursitis pain is through therapeutic imagery (see Chapter 6). Visualize the pain as a sword driven through your shoulder (or other painful area). As the sword is gradually drawn out and imaginary ice is applied to the painful area, the pain vanishes.

This, or a similar visualization, combined with the physical action-steps that follow, could form a powerful whole-person approach.

- *Step 1:* Apply cold for the first 48 hours. For the first 48 hours of the acute bursitis period, apply cold to the injured area. You can use a gel pack, a bag of crushed ice, or ice in a plastic bag. Cover with a towel and apply to the injured area for 30 minutes. Repeat 3 to 4 times a day until the pain and tenderness subside (or for a maximum of 48 hours after the injury occurs).

  If, as is often the case, the shoulder is the bursitis location, immobilize this joint by carrying the arm in a sling.

- *Step 2:* After the first 48 hours, apply moist heat. Once 48 hours has elapsed since the bursa injury, stop applying cold and begin to apply moist heat instead. Use a hot pack, a hot poultice, or a hot shower. A hot poultice made by wrapping a loaf of bread in a towel, soaking in very hot water, then wringing it out, is probably most effective. Apply heat for 20 minutes at a time, several times a day.

- *Step 3:* Use gentle exercise to restore movement. Before exercising, warm and stretch all muscles and tendons associated with the inflamed bursa. Apply moist heat as in step 2.

Once the acute stage ends and pain begins to subside, use gentle exercise to move and exercise the injured limb. The following exercises assume that bursitis occurred in the arm or shoulder (the most common location).

1. To prevent stiffness or atrophy, begin to swing the arm gently as soon as you can do so comfortably.
2. Hold on to the back of a chair and bend over at the waist to allow the painful arm and shoulder to hang down and swing loosely like a pendulum. Keeping the muscles relaxed, swing the arm from side to side, and then in ever-increasing circles.
3. As soon as you can, begin to raise both arms over your head. Try to stretch both arms up overhead several times a day. Keep reaching higher each day. If you cannot get your injured arm overhead, consider rigging a pulley so that, without ever hurting yourself, you

can pull your arm upward. Eventually, you will be able to raise your arm overhead without the pulley.

As normal movement is restored, add these additional movements.

4. Place a thick cushion or pad under the armpit of the injured shoulder. Keep the arm straight and allow it to hang down. Use your good arm to pull the elbow of the painful arm inward. This forces out the painful shoulder and relieves the pain.
5. Clasp your hands together behind your neck.
6. Clasp your hands behind your back. Then draw your elbows upward and toward each other. This alleviates pain by stretching the bursae in each shoulder.
7. Raise both arms straight overhead with palms facing to the rear. Bend both arms backward at the elbows and drop the hands so that the palms lie face down behind your shoulders. Repeat 5 times.
8. For this you'll need a chinning bar or a handy tree limb. Hold on to the bar and allow the body to hang loosely down. The resulting traction on the spine, shoulders, and elbows should help relieve bursitis pain in those areas.

PAINSTOPPER #33:
How to Relieve the Pain of Bursitis in the Hip

This technique was developed at the Mayo Clinic. It should not be used by anyone with a degenerative hip condition.

- *Step 1:* Stand erect and sideways to a wall with your painful hip next to the wall. You should be standing an arm's length from the wall.

- *Step 2:* Place your outside leg across and in front of the leg next to the wall. Keep both feet flat on the floor.

- *Step 3:* Support your body weight by placing your hand nearest the wall against the wall at shoulder height. Keep this supporting arm straight.

- *Step 4:* Gently roll your hips in toward the wall and back out again. Provided it is comfortable, you can continue to repeat this movement for 1 or 2 minutes. Repeat this step several times a day until the pain diminishes.

PAINSTOPPER #34:
Relieving the Pain of Tennis Elbow

Tennis elbow, the most common form of tendinitis, occurs when the tendons of the forearm muscle become strained. Microscopic tears in the tendon make the elbow tender and inflamed while pain extends along the upper side of the forearm. Swelling may also press on a nerve, causing pain to radiate to the shoulder and possibly to the wrist as well. The resulting pain may vary from mild to severe. It may be sporadic, or it may become constant and even disabling.

Tennis elbow is caused by repeated physical stress. The most common cause is improper backhand stroking in tennis. But golfers, rowers, and other exercisers may also experience tennis elbow. If it doesn't improve in a few days, you should see a doctor. The swelling *could* be due to a wrist fracture.

Treatment is similar to that for bursitis. During the first 48 hours, wrap an icepack around the elbow and forearm and secure with an elastic bandage. Keep the icepack in place for 30 minutes and reapply several times each day.

Alternatively, you can immerse your elbow in a bucket of ice-cold water for 30 minutes, or for as long as you can do so with reasonable comfort. Repeat several times a day during the 48 hours after injury occurs.

Once 48 hours has passed, stop applying cold and apply moist heat instead. Use the identical methods described in steps 1 and 2 of Painstopper #32: How to End Bursitis Pain. The injured arm should also be kept immobilized in a sling.

With this treatment, most cases of tennis elbow will subside spontaneously in about 30 days, even if you continue to play tennis. If the pain is bearable, you can probably continue to play while recovering. However, until recovery occurs, you are advised to use a two-handed backstroke. If pain occurs after playing, apply an icepack for 30 minutes several times a day until the pain lessens. Do not apply for longer than 48 hours after the pain recurs.

Once recovery is complete, you can easily prevent tennis elbow from recurring by strengthening the forearm and wrist muscles and by warming up and stretching for 10 minutes before beginning to actually play tennis or to row, and so on. It is also important to acquire a correct backhand stroke. Most tennis elbow results from jabbing at the ball instead of making a smooth, flowing, full-body backhand stroke. Keep your grip relaxed until the moment before you strike the ball.

- *Step 1:* Warm up and stretch before beginning to play. To prevent tennis elbow, warm up for a full 10 minutes before starting to exercise. Raise and stretch the arms repeatedly in every direction, especially overhead. As you do, continuously open and close the hands and fingers. Keep stretching until all joints feel warm and comfortable.

- *Step 2:* Kneel on a mat on the floor and place your hands on the floor about 10 inches in front of your kneecaps. Sit back on your heels. Keeping your palms facing down on the floor, turn your wrists so that your fingers are facing back toward your knees. This will stretch your wrists backward. Increase this stretch by gradually leaning forward so that you place more weight on your wrists. Although you will feel the stretch in your wrists, they should feel comfortable at all times. Avoid stretching past the point of comfort.

- *Step 3:* Stretch each wrist in the opposite direction. In this step, you curl the palm and fingers of one hand into a closed-fist position while bending the wrist down as far as you can. Meanwhile, use your other hand to apply mild pressure to increase the stretch. Repeat several times with each hand.

- *Step 4:* You can prevent a recurrence of tennis elbow by reinforcing your weakened forearm muscle. You'll need a light dumb-bell. Begin with 2 to 3 pounds. With palm facing up, support your forearm on a table or bench so that the wrist is over the edge and is free to move. Begin by slowly raising and lowering the wrist a dozen times in each direction. Then turn the arm over so that the palm faces down. Grasp the dumb-bell and slowly raise and lower it with your wrist. Do 10 repetitions. Rest for half a minute and repeat. As your muscle becomes stronger, add additional weight to maintain the same resistance. If a dumbbell is not available, place one or more cans of food in a plastic bag and hold the bag instead.

Several exercise physiologists have told me that this routine is just about the best and fastest way to end tennis elbow pain and to put an end to tennis elbow once and for all.

Chapter 10

NATURAL WAYS TO RELIEVE HEADACHE PAIN

For several years, Barbara N. had suffered from chronic migraine headaches. Only the most powerful vasoconstrictor drugs would help, and they left her feeling weak and nauseous for several days. But when she and her sister ordered chicken chow mein at a local Chinese restaurant, Barbara had no idea that a migraine attack would ruin her dinner.

The waiter had assured her that the chef would not use MSG. Yet just as she picked up her chopsticks, she felt the familiar throbbing pain. Within minutes, the pounding headache had enveloped her entire left eye and nostril.

Resignedly, she put down her chopsticks and dropped her head into her hands. "I'm sorry, I can't finish," she told the waiter. "I have a terrible migraine headache."

The waiter looked concerned. "Wait one moment," he said, "I'll get my father. He was born in China. He can show you a wonderful cure for headaches. It's called the Li-Shou method."

In under a minute, an elderly Chinese gentleman stood beside Barbara.

"Please to come to our spare room," he said, "I show how to stop migraine headache quickly with Chinese medicine."

Barbara was willing to try anything. She and her sister followed the restaurant owner into a vacant private dining room.

"Li-Shou work for all headache," he told Barbara. "Migraine. Tension. It stop them all."

He then showed Barbara a series of simple arm movements. As the final movement, Barbara was to swing her arms back and forth 100 times.

Incredibly, by the time she had completed 75 of the arm swings, Barbara realized that her migraine pain had disappeared.

She stopped in disbelief.

"It's incredible," she exclaimed. "The throbbing pain is completely gone."

"Ancient Chinese medicine better than modern drugs," the restaurant owner explained. "Do Li-Shou every day and you never have headache again."

The identical Li-Shou method that he taught Barbara is described step by step in Painstopper #35.

PAINSTOPPER #35:
Beat Headache Pain with Chinese Medicine

Here is how to practice the Chinese Li-Shou technique for swift relief of headache pain.

- *Step 1:* Stand upright with feet about 20 inches apart.

- *Step 2:* Rub the palms of your hands briskly together until they are warm.

- *Step 3:* Using your now-warm palms, lightly stroke your face from forehead to chin 30 times, always in the same direction. Stroke the flat of your face with your palms and avoid touching the eyes. Avoid rubbing or putting pressure on the face. Merely stroke your face lightly with your warm palms.

- *Step 4:* Remain standing in the original position with feet about 20 inches apart. Partially close your eyes and look down at your feet. Continue to hold this posture for the remainder of the exercise.

Extend your arms out in front, waist-high and with fingers touching.

Next, swing your arms back behind you until your fingers touch again. Then swing your arms out in front again until the fingers touch.

Keep swinging your arms from front to back and to front again, continuously and without stopping. Each complete swing from front to back and front again counts as one swing. Complete 100 of these arm-swings.

Throughout the arm swings, keep your eyes partially closed and continue to look down at your feet. Keep your awareness focused on your toes. If your thoughts wander off, bring your awareness back to your toes.

Chinese Medicine Stops Western Headaches

Li-Shou is Chinese for hand-swinging. Swinging the hands uses centrifugal force to shunt blood from swollen, dilated arteries in the head, and it directs the blood into the hands instead. As arteries in the hands dilate, more blood flows into the hands, making them warmer. The result is virtually identical to that achieved by biofeedback (see Painstopper #11). As blood is drawn from the head into the arms, the amount of blood flowing into the head diminishes.

Moreover, as you keep your awareness focused on your feet, blood vessels in the feet dilate, and more blood flows into the feet, making them warmer. And as a final benefit, the physical exercise of swinging the arms releases endorphin in the brain that blocks the experience of pain and helps to make you feel good instead.

Used according to these instructions, Li-Shou is highly effective at aborting either a migraine or tension headache that has already begun. To abort a migraine, you should begin to practice Li-Shou at the first hint of an approaching migraine or an aura (explained later).

Li-Shou is equally effective as a prophylactic to prevent headaches from occurring. After practicing Li-Shou once daily for about 3 weeks, arteries in the hands and feet remain fully or partially dilated throughout the day. This draws blood away from the head, making it impossible for blood vessels in the head to go into the explosive-dilation phase, the step that triggers most headache pain.

By practicing Li-Shou once each day, it becomes almost impossible for migraine to occur.

■ HOW HEADACHE PAIN OCCURS

Most headaches are either tension or migraine, and the underlying cause of both is unresolved emotional stress. In both types, the pain itself occurs as blood vessels in the head first overconstrict. As this cuts off the supply of oxygen to cells in the scalp, the cells send emergency signals for help. In a sudden rebound effect, blood vessels in the head and scalp then go into an explosive dilation. As artery walls are stretched, nerve endings literally scream with pain.

■ WHAT YOU SHOULD KNOW ABOUT TENSION HEADACHES

Tension (or muscle contraction) headaches are by far the most common type. Tension headache begins as stress is translated through the fight-or-flight response into abnormal contraction of the neck, shoulder, and scalp muscles. The same effect causes muscles surrounding each artery in the scalp and head to go into spasm. Immediately, the arteries become overconstricted, and the stage is set for a rebound dilation. It is this sudden dilation that causes the pain.

Tension-headache pain is a steady, relentless ache that travels up the back of the neck and around the ears, then spreads in a band around the head and forehead. After several hours, usually by evening, arteries begin to relax and the pain recedes. It may take 12 hours before a tension headache ends completely.

Most people tend to get acute tension headaches that are isolated and easily relieved by over-the-counter (OTC) drugs or natural therapies, and medical help is not required.

When emotional stress is unrelieved, it can provoke depression and anxiety and lead to chronic tension headaches. When tension headaches become chronic, they may continue without relief for months or years. A person with chronic tension headache lives in a continual stress-tension cycle. He or she wakes up with a tension headache and goes to bed with the same headache. Sleep is often disturbed and the victim wakes up feeling drowsy and fatigued. Drugs often provide only temporary relief, and the artery muscles in the scalp remain in a chronic state of spasm and contraction.

■ WHAT YOU SHOULD KNOW ABOUT MIGRAINE HEADACHES

Migraine headaches occur when emotional stress either triggers the fight-or-flight response or otherwise sets in motion a complex series of biochemical reactions that leads to overconstriction of arteries in the head. An explosive rebound dilation then occurs, stretching nerve endings and causing inflammatory responses in blood vessel walls that create the actual migraine pain.

The pain is intense and throbbing and is usually located on one side of the head only. Nausea and vomiting may occur, while hot flashes may alternate with shivering spells. Frequently, the victim must lie down in a darkened room until the pain ends. As the hours pass, the pounding pain becomes a steady ache. Eventually, sleep brings total relief and the migraine pain ends. But a sufferer often feels weak and washed out and may pass copious amounts of pale urine for several days afterward. Permanent physical damage is rare.

According to the National Center for Health Statistics, incidence of migraine is steadily rising, a trend believed due to the stress of modern living. Migraines are most common in women aged 20 to 40 and are believed to be linked with the time of menstruation and with the taking of estrogen and birth control pills.

Although the large-scale Harvard Physician's Health Study recently indicated that taking one aspirin every other day could reduce incidence of migraine by 20 percent, the standard treatment for migraine still consists of taking powerful drugs. Some of these drugs have such side effects as constriction of coronary arteries, while others may easily become addictive. Drugs are also used to prevent migraine attacks.

Roughly 20 percent of migraine victims experience the "classic" type of migraine headache, that is, a migraine preceded by a spectacular aura. An aura typically lasts for 10 – 30 minutes and includes visual disturbances and distortions of sense and perception. As the aura fades away, the hammering pain of migraine begins.

Most other migraine sufferers experience the "common" type of migraine headache that is not preceded by an aura.

Migraines are classified as vascular-type headaches. Most other vascular-type headaches are essentially migraines but are named for the trigger that sets them off. Thus we have ice cream headaches, exertion headaches, hangover headaches, hunger headaches, or menstrual headaches. The intensely painful cluster headache is also a vascular-type headache.

While emotional stress and physical tension set the stage for both classic and common migraine headaches, the headaches are actually set off by a variety of triggers. Migraine triggers range from certain foods to hunger or skipping meals; strenuous exercise; high altitudes; flickering or glaring lights, loud noises; hot, dry winds or weather; smoking or overindulgence in alcohol; oral contraceptives, excitement; abrupt changes of posture; certain medications; and dust, pollen, or pollution. Several of our action-steps focus on eliminating common migraine triggers.

The physical therapies in this chapter are primarily for use with either tension or migraine headaches. To make sure which type of headache you have, a medical examination is recommended. A physician can also identify whether your headache is disease related or benign. Statistics show that only 2 percent of headaches are disease related. So the risk that your headache is caused by a brain tumor, or other serious disease, is slight. Nonetheless, any new or more intense type of headache pain, or a change for the worse in your headache pattern, should prompt an early visit to a physician.

Once your headache has been diagnosed as a benign chronic headache, meaning it is not related to any specific disease, you can, with your physician's approval, begin to use any of the behavioral action-steps described in the remainder of this chapter.

■ A WHOLE-PERSON APPROACH RELIEVES HEADACHES BEST

Both chronic tension and migraine headaches can be permanently relieved, and future ones prevented, by using a whole-person approach in which one or more physical painstoppers described in this chapter is combined with the following painstoppers described in preceding chapters.

Painstopper #2: Walk Away from Pain

Painstopper #9: Relaxation Training—Nature's Prescription for Pain Relief

Painstopper #11: Biofeedback Training—Mind over Pain

Painstopper #21: Keep Pain at Bay with Positive Beliefs (including the Ten Affirmations That May Help Reduce Stress and Relieve Your Chronic Pain)

A combination of Painstoppers #9 and #11 is an excellent prophylactic for preventing either migraine or tension headache. Practice these action-steps three times daily; then gradually reduce to twice, then to once a day. Used together, Painstoppers #9 and #11 have also proved highly effective for aborting an approaching migraine or for relieving a migraine that has already begun.

PHYSICAL ACTION STEPS EFFECTIVE FOR BOTH TENSION AND MIGRAINE HEADACHES

PAINSTOPPER #36:
The One Best Natural Way to Stop and Prevent Headache Pain

The message of behavioral medicine is that we can change the way we feel by changing the way we act. When we feel the pain of a headache, we can usually change that feeling to one of comfort, provided we are willing to do something about it. Doing something about a headache is as simple as taking a brisk 35-minute walk, swim, or stationary bicycle ride.

Whether your headache is tension or migraine, brisk rhythmic exercise may alleviate it, or stop it altogether. And daily exercise may also prevent any further headaches. Tens of thousands of Americans have discovered that they can walk, swim, or pedal away almost any tension or migraine headache.

To alleviate a headache, you must walk, swim, or bicycle at a pace brisk enough to elevate your pulse and breathing rates. And the sign that this is happening is when you exercise briskly enough for perspiration to begin to appear on your brow. While walking, you can help to raise your pulse and breathing rates by swinging the arms vigorously up to shoulder height as you walk. However, you should never walk faster than will allow you to carry on a conversation.

Admittedly, most of us may not reach this level of activity during the first few exercise sessions. But in many cases, as little as 20 minutes of sufficiently brisk exercise has been enough to alleviate the pain of most migraine headaches by 50 percent or more.

■ EXERCISE PREVENTS ARTERY CONSTRICTION

Exercise is a powerful vasodilator. If begun soon enough, it prevents blood vessels in the head from reaching the intense state of constriction that sets the stage for a headache.

If the explosive dilation stage has already occurred, and the headache is in progress, exercise will help to normalize blood vessel diameter. Additionally, exercise releases endorphins in the brain that bind with pain receptors and prevent pain from being experienced.

Exercise therapy works best if you can begin at the first hint of an approaching tension or migraine headache. If possible, avoid the urge to lie down and begin to walk briskly instead, preferably outdoors. If this isn't possible, walk indoors or pedal a stationary bicycle (placed near an open window if conditions permit) or walk briskly up and down a flight of stairs or else swim at a brisk pace.

If your headache is so incapacitating that you simply cannot exercise, you should still recover sooner if you begin to exercise as soon as the pain allows it.

To overcome a headache, the exercise you choose must be brisk, rhythmic, and continuous and should, if possible, involve the body's largest muscle groups, such as the arms and legs. Stop-and-go exercises like baseball, doubles tennis, bowling, or golf create so little sustained oxygen uptake that they are almost useless for headache relief.

Naturally, you must be sufficiently fit to walk, swim, or bicycle briskly for 35 minutes. If you are not, and if you are over age 35, overweight, a smoker, a consumer of alcohol, or sedentary or unfit or have any disorder or dysfunction that may be worsened by exercise, you should consult your physician before beginning any type of exercise therapy. Or if you are a person for whom physical exertion is a migraine trigger, do not use exercise therapy for headache relief.

On the other hand, if you are already fit and enjoy brisk walking, you can walk (or do other exercise) for longer than 35 minutes. A walk of an hour or longer is even more beneficial.

For more information, turn back to Painstopper #2: Walk Away from Pain, and read it thoroughly.

PAINSTOPPER #37:
Stop Your Headache Cold—With Ice, Acupressure, and the Amazing Hoku Point

A cold pack may not be a panacea for every headache, but two recent studies have confirmed the effectiveness of this old-fashioned remedy. Carried out in 1986 at the Diamond Headache Clinic in Chicago, the first study observed the effect of icepack therapy on 90 patients who suffered from a variety of severe headaches, including migraine. The study revealed that when using coldpacks, 52 percent of patients experienced an immediate decrease in pain while 71 percent of all patients (including 80 percent of those with migraine) reported that coldpack therapy accelerated relief from headache pain.

A similar study by Robert Melzack at Canada's McGill University tested the effectiveness of coldpack therapy on 1,800 headache patients. The study found that 80 percent of patients experienced some degree of pain relief within 5 minutes. After applying the coldpack for a longer period, many patients with tension headaches reported complete pain relief.

In contrast, most migraine patients found that while coldpack therapy would abort an approaching migraine for an hour or more, additional coldpack applications were usually necessary to prevent a full-blown migraine headache from developing. The overall conclusion was that coldpack therapy would temporarily abort an approaching migraine or would provide partial relief for a migraine headache that had just begun. Coldpack therapy provided less benefit for a migraine headache that was already under way.

For a tension headache, apply a coldpack or gel pack for 15–20 minutes every hour until relief occurs. Cold is highly effective against mild-to-moderate tension headaches, less so against very severe tension headaches. Apply the coldpack to the most painful areas on your head.

For a migraine headache, place the coldpack against the forehead, eye, and nostril on the painful side of the face. If you can see any swollen, pulsating arteries, cover them with the icepack and keep it in place for up to 30 minutes. This should numb the arteries and cause them to constrict.

A coldpack can consist of a regular coldpack bag, or a plastic bag filled with crushed ice. Or you can use a cold gel pack. Wrap with a thin towel to prevent direct contact with skin.

For greater convenience, you may also consider Coldwrap®, a special headache coldpack that comes with an elastic headband and Velcro® closure and is available nowadays in most supermarkets and drugstores. The Coldwrap® is placed around the headband area and is tightened to minimize blood flow to the head.

How Hoku Halts Headaches

You can reinforce the effectiveness of cold therapy against either a tension or migraine headache by applying a single ice cube to your hoku acupressure point. The hoku point is at the apex of the web between thumb and forefinger. The exact location is in the fleshy part of the web immediately above where the bones of the thumb and forefinger meet.

Begin by massaging the hoku point of the hand on the same side as your headache pain. Hold an ice cube between the fingers and thumb of your other hand and massage the hoku point with a corner of the ice cube. Maintain steady pressure on the hoku point while you make small circular movements with the ice cube. Massage both sides of the thumb-forefinger web.

Then change over and massage the hoku point on your other hand. For best results, massage the hoku point while also applying a coldpack to your head. You can maintain the hoku point massage for 15–20 minutes. Use a new ice cube every few minutes.

PAINSTOPPER #38:
Close the Gate to Headache Pain

One reason that massage feels so good is that it stimulates the nervous system's fast fibers to close the body's pain gate. As you may recall from reading Chapter 2 (under the heading "Why Rubbing Takes the Ouch! Out of Pain"), you can often rub away pain by using self-massage. And you don't always have to rub or massage the painful area.

Frequently, rubbing a thumb will stop a headache as effectively as rubbing the scalp or forehead. The explanation is that neural stimulation from the thumb travels via fast nerve fibers and, when it reaches the pain gate, is given priority over pain impulses from a headache that travel via slow nerve fibers. The fast-fiber stimulation then overloads the pain gate controls, closing the pain gate and preventing headache pain impulses from reaching the brain.

The result? Headache pain is greatly reduced, or it cannot be felt at all.

You can close your pain gate to most headache pain by rubbing each of your thumbs vigorously for about 6 minutes apiece. Rub the top two joints of your right thumb briskly for 90 seconds. Then change over and rub the same two joints in your left thumb. Alternate every 90 seconds for a total of 12 minutes. Should your fingers and thumbs become sore, use baby oil or hand lotion as a lubricant.

Twelve minutes of active rubbing should relieve all but the most stubborn tension or migraine headache. If relief is only partial, continue rubbing for 6 more minutes. Since this action step does not actually stop a headache—it merely blocks pain impulses—you may have to repeat it several times.

PAINSTOPPER #39:
Brush Away Your Headache Pain

Imagine being able to brush away any headache with a few strokes of a hairbrush! It may sound like science fiction, but at many headache clinics, brushing is a proven therapy that is widely taught.

When he enrolled at a well-known Midwestern headache clinic, John W. not only learned to squelch his migraine headaches with relaxation and biofeedback, he was also taught how to brush away his headache pain.

The secret of brushing away a headache, John learned, is to constantly rotate the brush against the scalp using a circular motion. Rotate the brush in circles about half an inch in diameter so that the upper part of the circular motion always moves toward the back of the head.

Then, while maintaining this rotary motion, John was taught to brush his hair in a special way. His first brush stroke always begins above his left eyebrow. From there, he moves the brush up and over his temple to the scalp. Next, he dips the brush down in front of his left ear until the center of the brush is level with his earlobe. Without interrupting the rotary motion, he then moves the brush upward in front of his left ear and back over the top of the ear. The brush stroke then continues on back across the scalp, and it finally drops down to the back of the neck.

By taking this path, John's brush applies a brisk, rotary massage to both his temporal and occipital arteries, relaxing their muscles and restoring the blood vessels to their normal diameter.

John's next brush stroke begins 1 inch to the right of the previous stroke and follows a parallel path 1 inch above it. John begins each successive brush stroke 1 inch higher until finally he brushes straight back over the center and crown of his head and down the center of his neck.

At this point, he begins the entire process on the other side of his head.

Your Hairbrush—A Natural Analgesic

After learning the brush strokes and practicing for a few days, John was able to brush his entire scalp in under 2 minutes. Whenever he feels a migraine approaching, he immediately begins to brush his scalp. Almost always, the migraine is aborted. To ensure that the migraine does not return, he repeats the brushing routine at 30-minute intervals for 2 or 3 hours.

John can also brush away a full-blown migraine headache should one occur. The first brushing usually cuts the intensity of the pain by half. A few minutes later, John gives his scalp another brushing. And 15 minutes later, he brushes his scalp again. By this time, the headache is usually gone.

John also uses his brushing routine 3 times a day as a prophylactic against possible future migraine attacks.

John recommends using a moderately stiff, natural-fiber hairbrush. Should he not have his hairbrush handy when a headache seems imminent, he duplicates his hairbrush routine by using his fingers. Since a scalp massage with the fingers is not as efficient as using a brush, he repeats each finger "brush" stroke a second time.

Experiments at headache clinics show that brushing therapy is equally effective on either tension or migraine headaches. After a brushing session is completed, allow about 15 minutes for pain relief to appear. Brushing is more effective on migraines if you begin the brush strokes at the first indication of an impending headache.

For brushing to work, the scalp must be dry. Some women's hair styles may also conceivably interfere with brushing. And in some migraine victims, the scalp becomes so sensitive during a headache that brushing is impossible.

Yet as John discovered, brushing remains one of the simplest and most successful ways to relieve a headache naturally.

PAINSTOPPER #40:
Prevent Headache Pain with a Facial Tone-up

Poor muscle tone in face and head muscles is frequently duplicated in the smooth muscles that surround every artery in the head. Poor tone in blood vessel muscles allows the abnormal constriction and dilation that causes headache pain.

Researchers at several pain clinics have found that when muscles in the head and face are toned-up by exercise, the tone of artery muscles also improves. Blood vessels are then able to normalize their diameter instead of becoming excessively constricted and, later, excessively dilated.

Results from several pain and headache clinics show that toning up the facial muscles twice a day almost invariably leads to a significant decrease in the frequency and intensity of both chronic tension and migraine headaches. Toning up the facial muscles may also bring swift relief for a headache that has already begun.

- *Step 1:* To tone your facial muscles, tense all the muscles in your face, forehead, and scalp as tightly as possible. Hold for 6 seconds; then release. Be certain that you include every part of every muscle. Then repeat the exercise 9 more times (for a total of 10 times).

- *Step 2:* Using your eye muscles only, squeeze your eyes tightly shut. Hold 6 seconds, and release. Then open your eyes as wide as possible; hold 6 seconds, and release. Raise the eyebrows and look up as high as you can; hold 6 seconds and release. Then look down as far as you can; hold 6 seconds, and release.

- *Step 3:* Next, for exactly 60 seconds, make faces, frown, smile, wiggle your ears and scalp, yawn, wrinkle your nose, and have a hearty laugh.

Hundreds of Americans have learned to use these action-steps twice daily to prevent or relieve most types of chronic tension or migraine headaches.

PHYSICAL ACTION STEPS PRIMARILY EFFECTIVE FOR TENSION HEADACHES

PAINSTOPPER #41:
Soak Away Tension Headaches

A long soak in a hot tub bath often works wonders in dispelling a persistent tension headache.

- *Step 1:* Fill the bath with water that is as hot as you can stand without discomfort. As soon as you turn on the faucet, and while the bath is filling, begin the following relaxation exercises.

- *Step 2:* Do a series of neck rolls, followed by raising and lowering the shoulders, and rotating the shoulders with a circular motion. Yawn several times. Then get into the bath. You can scent the bath with peppermint oil, which has a relaxing aroma.

- *Step 3:* After relaxing in the tub for a few minutes, begin to gently raise and rotate your shoulders and to move and swing your arms. Stretch your neck in all directions and yawn again several times.

- *Step 4:* Stay in the bath until your neck and shoulder muscles feel completely relaxed. Then get out and towel yourself dry.

- *Step 5:* If you still have a headache, lie down and place a cold gel or ice pack over the painful area. Within a few minutes, all traces of any tension headache should have disappeared.

PAINSTOPPER #42:
Shower Away Your Tension Headache

By directing the spray from your shower on to the back of your head, neck, shoulders, and upper back, you can relieve most tension headaches in a matter of minutes.

- *Step 1:* Stand under a shower and turn on the water until it is as warm as you can stand without discomfort. Direct the spray on your back, neck, shoulders, and scalp for at least 5 minutes. Meanwhile, massage the muscles in these areas with your hands, or have someone else give you a massage.

- *Step 2:* When you feel thoroughly soothed and relaxed, turn the faucet so that cool, brisk water flows over the same areas. Run the water as cool as you can without discomfort or shocking the body. Limit exposure to the cool shower to a maximum of 4 minutes.

- *Step 3:* By the time you towel yourself dry, the average tension headache should have disappeared. If you wish, you can repeat the cycle.

Alternative applications of heat followed by cold relieve tension headaches by releasing stored-up tension in taut neck and shoulder muscles. If you haven't time to take a shower, try leaning back in an easy chair and draping a hot, moist towel over the back of your neck. Then massage the scalp, neck, and shoulder muscles.

PAINSTOPPER #43:
Massage Away Your Tension Headache

Most tension headaches are due to muscle contraction in the neck and shoulders. You can relieve most tension headaches by massaging these muscles until they relax. The headache should then begin to subside.

For best results, sit at a table. Support your forehead with the left hand so that the elbow is on the table. Using the thumb and fingers of the right hand, begin to knead and massage the muscles at the back of the neck. Use a circular motion as you squeeze and work over your tense neck muscles. Use your knuckles and fingers to give your scalp a vigorous massage.

To avoid fatigue, change hands every 60 seconds. Without actually hurting yourself or causing any discomfort, dig your fingers into your neck and shoulder muscles and give them a vigorous massage. Work up and down your entire musculature, from the trapezius muscles in your shoulders to the top of your scalp, several times.

Usually, it takes only 5 or 6 minutes to relax the muscles, and your headache should begin to fade soon afterward.

You may also press and massage the forehead, headband area, or temples, wherever a headache is located. Simple as it sounds, merely pressing on painful areas of the head or temples with the palms and fingers, is a highly effective way to temporarily relieve headache pain (including migraine).

During a migraine attack, you may also see blood vessels on the forehead that are visibly bloated, pulsating, or distended. By applying steady pressure to the blood vessel area, the headache pain almost always diminishes.

As you maintain steady pressure on a painful area, you can also impart a circular motion with your palms or fingers. This rubbing movement creates fast-fiber stimulation, which helps your pain gate to close. Applying light but firm massage to the site of headache pain also helps to normalize muscle tone. In turn, this reduces the excessive dilation of blood vessels in the headache area.

PAINSTOPPER #44:

Easy Stretching May Provide Permanent Relief for Tension Headaches

Back in the 1980s. a group of neurologists discovered that taut neck muscles were the mechanical cause of most tension headaches. In response, they developed a series of neck-stretching exercises that proved extraordinarily successful in permanently relieving most chronic tension headaches.

Studies at several headache clinics have shown that, after practicing neck-stretching exercises for six weeks, 50 percent of participants reported complete freedom from chronic tension headaches. After practicing neck-stretching exercises daily for three months, virtually everyone in the studies reported complete relief. Only a few of the most stubborn cases showed no improvement.

Other surveys have confirmed that neck stretching provides fast relief for acute tension headache—the occasional headache that millions experience daily. Neck stretching has also helped some people with common migraine headaches.

The exercises consist of exerting gentle pressure with the hands to stretch and release taut muscles and fibers in the neck. To do the stretches, sit upright in a chair.

- *Step 1:* Turn your head to the right as though looking back over your right shoulder.

- *Step 2:* Place your right index finger under your left cheek so that your palm and thumb are under your chin. Exert gentle pressure to push your head around to the right.

- *Step 3:* Place the left hand on top of your head so that the tip of your middle finger touches your right ear. Then exert gentle pressure to pull your head down toward your chest.

  Ease up on the pressure immediately if you begin to feel discomfort. Back off slightly, and then hold at this point for 10 seconds. Then release.

- *Step 4:* Repeat steps 1, 2, and 3 on the other side of your head.

- *Step 5:* Repeat the stretch twice more on each side of your head, making a total of six stretches, three on each side. Then lower your hands and relax your neck.

- *Step 6:* Raise both shoulders as if trying to touch your earlobes. Hold 15 seconds, and release.

- *Step 7:* Raise your chin as high as you can while you drop your head back as far as you can. Hold 15 seconds, and release.

- *Step 8:* Lower your head on to your chest and stretch your neck as far forward as you can. Hold 15 seconds, and release.

- *Step 9:* Take six deep, abdominal breaths, filling the belly with air first and the upper chest last. Exhale fully and at leisure. (Abdominal breathing is described in Painstopper #7.)

This routine quickly releases stress and tension in the neck muscles, and it can be done almost anywhere. Apply steady, gentle pressure and stop at the point where mild discomfort appears. Discontinue altogether if you experience any discomfort, pain, or dizziness.

After a day or two of practice, you should be able to complete the entire routine in under 4 minutes. To relieve chronic tension headache, perform one series of stretches (steps 1 to 9) every two hours during the day. Once the headache pain disappears, continue to do one series of stretches twice a day as a prophylactic.

PHYSICAL ACTION-STEPS PRIMARILY EFFECTIVE FOR MIGRAINE HEADACHES

PAINSTOPPER #45:
Banish Headaches with "Instant Biofeedback"

Immersing the hands and feet in very warm water may abort or stop a migraine headache almost as effectively as biofeedback. While biofeedback warms the hands and feet by training the mind to dilate arteries, you can warm your hands and feet even more rapidly by placing them in very warm water.

To get started, you'll need a small footbath or a bucket large enough to immerse both feet above the ankles. At the same time, you must immerse both hands above the wrists in another bucket or washbasin. Some migraine sufferers report good results by filling a tub bath to a depth of 7 inches and then sitting in the tub on a stool about 12 inches high. With their ankles already immersed, they then lean forward and immerse their hands to above the wrists.

Most people find that water at 111° Fahrenheit warms very effectively without causing discomfort. If using a footbath or buckets, keep a hot-water faucet running slowly so that you can refill the bucket with hot water to maintain the temperature.

Whether you use biofeedback or warm water to warm the extremities, the effect is similar. Warming the hands and feet causes arteries to dilate. This increases blood flow into the hands and feet, making them still warmer. The same process draws blood away from arteries in the head that have become bloated and stretched by the migraine sequence. Within 15–20 minutes, most head arteries tend to return to normal size. As a result, either the headache pain is significantly diminished, or the migraine has been aborted altogether.

Warming the extremities with water is a temporary expedient that must be repeated again at each onset of a migraine headache. The warming effect never becomes semipermanent as it does when biofeedback training is practiced regularly.

For long-lasting prevention of migraine headaches, learning to use biofeedback is worth the extra time and effort. Biofeedback is also one of the best stress-reducing action-steps around.

PAINSTOPPER #46:
Head Off Your Headache with Heat

You can often abort an impending migraine if you can apply heat to the scalp in time Those with classic migraine are usually alerted to the approach of a headache when the aura begins. But even if you suffer from common migraine (which is not preceded by an aura), subtle feelings or vague symptoms may still alert you to an approaching headache.

In either case, if you immediately begin to apply warmth to the scalp, you can usually head off an upcoming migraine. Should the headache still materialize, the pain is almost always milder and more subdued.

The quickest way to apply heat is with a bonnet-type hairdryer. While these traditional hairdryers have been replaced in recent years by blower-type dryers, the bonnet type can still be found.

Use the "warm" setting. At the first hint of an approaching migraine, turn on the bonnet-dryer and sit under it. Alternatively, try using a heating pad set on "low." But it must cover the scalp, so secure it with a headband or belt.

Lacking a hairdryer or heating pad, apply heat to the scalp with a hot pack or hot compress, or even with a towel wrung out in hot water. Use the hot pack to cover as much of the scalp as possible, and drape any surplus down the back of the neck. Dip the pack in hot water and wring out at intervals to maintain heat.

Another alternative is to use a hot shower to apply heat to the scalp. At the first hint of an approaching migraine, get under the shower and spray the scalp, forehead, and neck with warm-to-hot water. Use only warm water and do not alternate with a cold spray.

Regardless of how you apply heat to the scalp, once the headache appears to have been aborted, remove the heat and massage the scalp with your fingers. Use a circular motion and work down to the ears and back of the neck.

As you have probably guessed, warmth prevents a migraine from manifesting by dilating arteries in the head during the constriction phase of the migraine sequence. In this way, the arteries are prevented from undergoing the explosive dilation that creates the migraine pain.

Once a migraine headache actually begins, you should stop applying heat to the scalp. It's too late. The explosive dilation has already occurred, and the migraine is well under way.

As usual, whenever applying heat or cold, the temperature should always remain in the comfort zone, and extremes of temperature should be avoided. Anyone with diabetes, or any other dysfunction that may distort the sensation of heat or cold, should not use heat or cold therapy for any type of pain relief without medical supervision.

PAINSTOPPER #47:
A Simple Food That May Phase Out Migraine Headaches

It doesn't work for everyone. But headache literature reveals that many women who suffer from chronic migraine headaches have been able to prevent further headaches by increasing their intake of vitamins B3 and C and the mineral magnesium.

Two independent university studies have each shown that four out of five Americans are deficient in magnesium reserves and that these deficiencies may directly trigger chronic migraine headaches.

At Eastern Tennessee State University, 500 women with chronic migraine headaches were given either a 100-mg or 200 mg supplement of magnesium each day. Within hours, some women began reporting headache relief. After several days, over half the women reported greatly diminished headache pain. Several women who had suffered unbroken headache pain for over two weeks became symptom-free. Seventy percent of the 500 women migraineurs remained completely free of headaches for as long as they continued taking the magnesium supplements.

A similar study at Case Western Reserve found that 80 percent of women migraine sufferers became symptom-free after taking 200-mg of magnesium daily for three weeks. One woman in the study, who had suffered a weekly migraine attack for over ten years, was unable to stop her headaches with drugs. She was constantly sick with pain and depression. But after taking 200 mg of magnesium daily for 28 days, her headaches had almost completely disappeared.

The consensus of medical opinion is that magnesium relaxes the smooth muscles that enclose the arteries causing them to dilate. Thus magnesium blocks the migraine process.

Supplements containing 200 mg of magnesium are available in a variety of forms at health food stores and at many supermarkets and drugstores. While you should consult your physician before taking magnesium supplements if you have any kidney or other health problem, or are taking medication, an intake of 200 mg per day is considered risk-free by most nutritionists.

You can also increase magnesium uptake by eating avocados, nuts, or peas or beans. Beware, however, of caffeinated sodas, alcohol, or certain medications. Each of these may bind with magnesium and prevent its absorption into the body.

Low B-Vitamin Levels Linked to Migraine Headaches in Women

Several prominent clinical ecologists (allergy specialists) have reported finding consistently low levels of B vitamins in chronic migraine patients, almost always in women. After these women were placed on a diet high in B vitamins and vitamin C, the majority found that their headaches began to gradually disappear.

The best way to add B vitamins and vitamin C to the diet is to eat many more helpings of fruits, vegetables, and whole grains than is customary in the standard American diet. And the best single food source of B vitamins is probably brewer's yeast, available inexpensively in all health food stores.

As a headache prophylactic, add 2–3 heaping tablespoons of brewer's yeast to your breakfast cereal, or stir 2 tablespoons into a glass of fresh orange juice each morning. Obviously, if yeast is a migraine trigger food for you, you should never add brewer's yeast to your food.

Supplements Work Too

You can take a B-complex supplement that contains all B vitamins as well as B3. I recommend your taking a supplement that contains *all* B complex vitamins rather than B3 alone. The reason is that B vitamins are more effective when the entire complex is taken together.

Supplements containing 100 mg of the most important B vitamins are available at supermarkets and health food stores, and the manufacturer's recommendation is usually to take one tablet per day, preferably with meals. Most people can safely take supplementary B vitamins and vitamin C, in moderate amounts. However, if you have any condition or dysfunction that might be affected by taking vitamin supplements, you should consult your physician before taking them.

If you eat fewer than four servings of fruit and five servings of vegetables per day, you will probably also benefit by taking 500 mg of supplemental vitamin C daily.

Most case histories show that it takes two to three weeks to notice any decrease in headache frequency. Many women take vitamin and mineral supplements for six weeks before noticing any significant results. Gradually, however, incidence of migraine attacks is likely to decrease, and in many cases, the headaches disappear altogether.

It's worth noting that diets low in B vitamins and vitamin C are invariably diets high in meats, fat, and refined carbohydrates (white flour and sugar) and deficient in fruits, vegetables, legumes, and whole grains.

Such a diet may also lead to heart disease, cancer, and other chronic diseases. You will also read (in Painstopper #48) that Temple University researchers discovered that a plant-based diet significantly helped to reduce, or even eliminate, migraine pain.

Hilda L. Nullifies Migraine with Niacin

Now this is strictly an anecdote and has not been confirmed by any study or observation. But a woman friend, Hilda L., swears she can abort an impending classic migraine by taking 50 mg of vitamin B3 in the form of niacin. (Vitamin B3 is available either in the form of niacin or as niacinamide.) Hilda takes the niacin at the first hint of an approaching aura. Apparently, the niacin dilates blood vessels in the head during the constriction phase of the migraine sequence. This interrupts the migraine process, and the headache is aborted.

Since niacin must be taken at least 20 minutes before onset of the migraine headache, it is effective only against classic migraine. Some 20 – 30 minutes before a classic migraine strikes, it is preceded by an aura. The aura was Hilda's warning to take the niacin.

Vitamin B3 is available in two forms: niacin, which dilates capillaries and causes a skin flush, and niacinamide, which does not. Apparently, only niacin has been found to abort an impending migraine. For prophylactic use, however, niacinamide is just as effective and does not cause a skin flush. (Caution: niacin should not be used for cluster headaches.)

PAINSTOPPER #48:
How to Identify Foods That May Be Causing Your Migraine Headaches

In recent years, several landmark studies have confirmed that migraine headaches are commonly triggered by eating certain foods. These foods are known as migraine trigger foods.

One study at London's Charing Cross Hospital examined the effects of various trigger foods on 60 chronic migraine patients. When the most common trigger foods were eliminated, 50 of the 60 participants in the study became headache-free.

The Ten Most Common Migraine Trigger Foods

Corn and wheat products

Chocolate and chocolate milk

All whole-milk products, especially yellow and aged cheeses

Any meat, fish, or vegetable that is processed, pickled, salted, smoked, cured, aged, marinated, or fermented (including ham, bacon, hot dogs, and all sausages, pickled herring, or caviar)

Alcoholic beverages, especially certain beers and aged or red wines

MSG (monosodium glutamate)

Yeast and yeast products, including bread made with yeast

Beef, pork, or liver

Eggs

Certain seafoods and shellfish

Another recent study of patients with migraine by researchers at Temple University in Philadelphia tested the migraine trigger effects of various diets. The study revealed that it is primarily foods of animal origin that are migraine triggers, and the reason is that all are exceptionally high in amino acids. While corn and wheat, and especially refined wheat (white flour), are commonly migraine trigger foods, and tomatoes, onions, nuts, beans, and olives occasionally trigger migraines, most plant-based (vegetarian) foods do *not* set off migraine headaches.

Many vegetarians have told me that after adopting an exclusively plant-based diet, their migraine headaches disappeared. This same finding was confirmed by the Temple University study. Researchers there discovered that a plant-based diet low in animal protein, fats, and refined carbohydrates (white flour and sugar) significantly helped to reduce, or even to eliminate, migraine pain.

Among other foods that the researchers identified as potential migraine triggers were all fats and oils, fried foods, butter and margarine, fatty meats, white flour, sugar and sweeteners (including frozen fruit juices with sugar added), nondairy creamers, and preserves, jellies, coffee and caffeinated sodas, baked goods, pies, brownies, doughnuts, cookies, cakes, and candies. Many canned, manufactured, and preserved foods also contain migraine triggers.

The principal migraine triggers are amino acids such as tyramine, phenylalanine, and octapamine plus the sodium nitrates and nitrites commonly found in cured meats. All these are potent vasodilators. When eaten during the evening and early night hours, these foods can trigger neurological mechanisms that dilate arteries in the head and set off the migraine sequence.

Foods That Rarely Trigger Migraines

Among foods least likely to trigger a migraine attack in the average person are bran muffins; brown rice; all cooked and dry whole-grain breakfast cereals that are free of corn, wheat, or sugar; homemade vegetable soups or stews; melons; mixed vegetable juices; fresh fruits (except citrus, bananas, tomatoes, avocadoes, plums, and prunes); puffed rice; fresh unsweetened fruit juices; raw seeds; rice and rice flour; and tapioca.

Most cooked vegetables (excluding peas, beans, and onions) when steamed, or baked in a casserole, are also unlikely to give rise to a migraine. Small helpings of chicken or fish are also seldom migraine triggers. Such foods should always be boiled, broiled, baked, or steamed, never fried.

Perhaps we should not be too surprised to learn that the majority of foods that do *not* provoke migraines are the same foods that do *not* provoke heart disease, cancer, osteoporosis, diabetes, and other degenerative diseases that eventually kill off most Americans (see Painstopper #3: The One Diet That Does It All).

Identifying the Food That Is Triggering Your Migraine

If you eat a diet composed exclusively of these migraine-safe foods for ten days, and your migraines continue as usual, all indications are that your migraines are *not* caused by any migraine trigger food. In this case, you can safely return to your normal diet.

However, if your migraine headaches diminish or disappear, they could very well be triggered by one or more of the foods you normally eat.

One way to identify the exact migraine trigger food that is causing your headaches is to introduce back into your diet, one by one, the ten most common migraine trigger foods listed earlier.

Before you do, however, make a list of the three foods you crave the most and that you are always eating. If one or more coincide with the ten most common migraine trigger foods, consider these foods as your prime suspects.

You should now test each of these foods by using an elimination diet. To begin testing, continue to eat your migraine-safe diet, but make each meal about 15 percent smaller than usual. Replace this missing 15 percent with a normal-size helping of the suspect food you are testing. Keep this up for 48 hours. If the suspect food actually is a migraine trigger, it should provoke a reaction within this time. If not, then go on to test your second most suspect food in the same way.

Once a suspect food has failed to provoke a headache during a 48-hour testing period, you can add it back into your diet. As a general rule, you should not test more than four foods consecutively. After testing four foods, return to your normal diet. Wait for a week or so. Then begin testing once more from the start.

A stockbroker acquaintance of mine, Stuart B., was recently plagued by debilitating migraine headaches and fatigue. While preparing this book, I let him read the copy in Painstopper #48. Stuart immediately went on a migraine-safe diet and ten days later began to test the foods he suspected most. After testing four foods, he found he was sensitive to eggs and cured meats.

Stuart may not have identified all his migraine trigger foods yet. But he has already cut in half the severity and frequency of his chronic migraine headaches.

PAINSTOPPER #49:
An Herb That Often Ends or Alleviates Migraine Pain

Several well-documented studies in Britain have concluded that the herb feverfew, taken prophylactically, may prevent migraine attacks. And if a migraine does develop, the pain is significantly diminished.

Feverfew is a plant of the chrysanthemum, or daisy, family. Participants in the British studies either ate a few leaves of fresh or freeze-dried feverfew each day, or they took supplement capsules containing feverfew.

In a double-blind study at the City of London Migraine Clinic (reported in the *British Medical Journal,* August 31, 1985), participants who took feverfew for an extended period reported an average of only 1.5 migraine headaches per month compared to 3.4 per month in the control group. In another study at the same clinic, 30 percent of those taking feverfew reported complete cessation of migraine attacks while 70 percent reported fewer attacks and less pain.

In yet another study at the University of Nottingham, a group taking feverfew in capsule form reported an average 24 percent reduction in the number of headaches, while the severity and symptoms of the headaches, such as vomiting and nausea, was considerably less (reported in *Lancet*, July 23, 1988).

What Makes Feverfew Work

British researchers believe that the active ingredients in feverfew are parthenolide and sesquiterpene-lactone. These agents inhibit release of the neurotransmitter serotonin, a potent vasoconstrictor, into the bloodstream. Without sufficient serotonin, arteries in the head are unable to enter the excessive-constriction phase, an essential step in the migraine sequence. As a result, a migraine headache cannot occur.

Based on these studies, feverfew appears equally effective whether the leaves are eaten fresh, or freeze dried, or in the form of nutritional capsules. Most study participants ate either one large feverfew leaf daily or two medium-sized leaves or three or four smaller ones.

To mask the herb's bitter, camphor-like taste, most participants preferred to eat the yellow-green leaves between two pieces of whole-wheat bread spread with honey. Those taking capsules consumed two 50 mg capsules per day. However, most Britons who take feverfew report improved results by taking three capsules daily.

Feverfew capsules sold in U.S. health food stores usually contain 340 mg per capsule and the manufacturer's recommended daily dose may vary from one to three capsules. This appears to be considerably more than the dosage used in the British studies. And it is hoped, it produces even better results.

While in England, I was told that capsules made of freeze-dried feverfew leaves were more effective than those made with sun-dried leaves. Apparently, heat of any kind may destroy the active ingredients in the leaves.

Some health food stores may also stock feverfew in tincture or tablet form. Tablets should be swallowed with a glass of water to avoid the bitter taste. Dried feverfew leaves may also be available as an herb tea. One herbalist told me that steeping three-fourths of a teaspoon of the tea in a cup of boiling water should give the right strength. As a migraine prophylactic, you can drink 3 cups of feverfew tea daily. Tea can also be made from feverfew capsules.

Only Authentic Feverfew Will Do

Regardless of the form in which you take feverfew, genuine feverfew should bear the botanical name *Chrysanthemum parthenum*. Anything else may not work.

Even with genuine feverfew, don't expect immediate results. To work effectively, feverfew must be taken daily and over an extended period. Feverfew may also have some minor side effects.

Eighteen percent of British users who consumed feverfew in leaf form experienced allergic reactions in the tongue and mouth. Direct contact with the leaves also caused several cases of mouth ulcers (which disappeared when the feverfew was stopped). Most pharmacists consider that feverfew has about the same toxicity, and is about as addictive, as coffee. For instance, after long-term use, some Britons reported withdrawal symptoms such as joint stiffness, nervousness, or sleeplessness.

Feverfew should not be taken by pregnant women or by anyone allergic to ragweed. In some people, it can lower blood pressure, increase appetite, or cause diarrhea. Again, feverfew has not helped every migraine sufferer nor have its long-term effects been completely studied. For these reasons, feverfew is best taken under the supervision of a naturopath or other licensed health professional.

Chapter 11

NATURAL WAYS TO RELIEVE LOWER BACK PAIN

You've just been hit by acute lower back pain! The pain is agonizing, like being stabbed in the small of the back with a knife. You stand frozen, not daring to move, holding on to a chair for support.

What to do next?

Almost always, acute back pain is due to a muscle spasm. You've torn a tiny piece of tissue in a lower back muscle. To protect against further movement, the area around the injury has gone into spasm. The spasm then exerts pressure on adjacent nerve endings, causing the pain.

Your immediate concern is to relieve the pain. To do that, you must relieve the spasm. Pain or not, you're going to have to move, even if it's only to reach the nearest couch.

So let's get started by carrying out the action-steps in Painstopper #50.

PAINSTOPPER #50:
How to Relieve Acute Back Pain

Your immediate need is to give your back muscles a chance to rest and relax.

189

- *Step 1:* Get into bed and take two aspirin or ibuprofen to relieve pain and inflammation. According to several prominent back specialists, you can often speed recovery at this point if, before getting into bed, you lie on your back on a rug or carpet on the floor beside the bed (or a chair). Then raise your legs and bend the knees so that your calves and feet are resting on the bed or chair. Keep your head, shoulders, and spine flat on the floor. Place a thin pillow or folded towel under your head for support. The back specialists all agreed that if you can adopt this position within a few minutes of first experiencing lower back pain, the pain may either soon disappear or be much less severe. Hold this position for 20 – 30 minutes if you can. Then get into bed.

- *Step 2:* If pain persists, begin applying cold to the painful area. Use a cold gel pack or icebag or a plastic bag filled with ice cubes. Cover with a single layer of thin towel to protect the skin. Keep the coldpack on for as long as you feel a burning sensation.

  Immediately after your back is numb, remove the coldpack. In any case, do not apply the coldpack for longer than 15–20 minutes at a time. For as long as pain persists, reapply the coldpack for up to 20 minutes once every 3 hours. After each application, your back should be numb and pain-free. If, after 24 hours of application, cold has not relieved the pain, then stop applying cold and begin applying heat as in step 3.

- *Step 3:* Either cold or heat, or a combination of both, may dilate blood vessels in the back, allowing more oxygen and nutrients to reach muscle cells and end the spasm.

  Always begin by applying cold to the injury for the first 24 hours. After 24 hours, if pain still persists, stop applying cold and begin to apply moist heat to the spasm area.

  To apply moist heat, simply take a hot soak in a tub bath for 30 minutes at a time. You can take a maximum of four hot tub baths each day.

  If you cannot get in and out of a tub, apply a hot pack consisting of a moist towel covered by a layer of plastic to keep the heat in. Or better, use a hot compress made by wrapping a loaf of bread in a towel, soaking it in hot water, wringing it out, and then wrapping it in a layer of plastic to keep in the heat.

Apply the hot pack to the spasm area for 20–30 minutes at a time for a maximum of 4 times each day. Another possible alternative is to stand under a warm-to-hot shower and spray the painful area for 20–30 minutes with a maximum of four showers per day. If you cannot apply moist heat, use a heating pad set on "low" or "medium." Place a single layer of thin towel between the pad and the skin. And place a light, folded blanket over the pad to keep in the heat.

However you apply heat, do not remain immobile for more than 30 minutes at a time. After being in one position for 30 minutes, change your position and try to move around. To get out of bed with a painful back, roll on your side and push yourself up with your arms.

As you experience some degree of pain relief, begin to move as much as you can. Move your arms and legs to limber up. Stretch as much as possible. If you can do so without pain, bend your spine forward and arch it back.

- *Step 4:* If, 48 hours after injury occurred, pain still persists, many back specialists have recommended applying contrasting heat and cold to the spasm area.

The simplest way is to stand under a shower as warm as you can comfortably stand for 10 minutes. Spray the water over the spasm area. As you do, partially bend your knees and place your hands on your thighs just above your knees. Hold this position as the warm water soothes your aching back. Then raise your right hip, move it back, and return to normal position. Repeat with the left hip. Maintain this exercise for several minutes as you continue to enjoy the warm, relaxing spray.

Then switch to a cool, brisk shower for 2 minutes. The cool shower should not be so cold as to shock the body or to induce any actual discomfort.

Repeat the entire hot and cold shower routine one more time. Finally, end up with a few minutes under the warm water spray. Towel briskly dry and relax in a warm bed for half an hour.

Limit the use of contrasting hot and cold showers to a maximum of 4 times each day. You should not need to continue using contrasting hot-cold showers after the evening of the fourth day following the injury.

- *Step 5:* As soon as you are able, begin to do the pelvic tilt (see Painstopper #52).

  Briefly, you lie flat on your back in bed with knees raised, heels drawn in toward your buttocks, and arms stretched out sideways. Inhale deeply, filling the belly with air. At the same time, arch the back so that your weight is on the buttocks. Then, as you exhale, tighten your abdominal and buttock muscles and press the small of your back flat onto the bed. Simultaneously, suck in your abdomen and rock the pelvis forward, giving the back muscles a magnificent stretch and releasing the spasm.

  Provided there is no discomfort, you can repeat the pelvic tilt exercise several times a day, and you can do more repetitions each time.

- *Step 6:* As your back pain gradually subsides, repeat the pose in step 1. That is, lie on the floor beside the bed on a rug or carpet and support your head with a low pillow or folded towel. Bend your knees and raise your legs so that your feet and calves are on the bed. Keep your head, shoulders, and spine flat on the floor. Remain in this position for up to 30 minutes. You can repeat this exercise up to 4 times a day.

- *Step 7:* Massage is another wonderful way to help your back to recover. If you cannot persuade anyone to massage your back, try this self-massage technique.

  Lie on your back on a rug on the floor. Then slide one tennis ball under each side of your spine in your painful small-of-the-back area. Next gently move your body so that the balls work up, down, and around the painful area, giving your back a deep-pressure massage.

  Golf balls will often work if tennis balls are unavailable. If you like, you can also place two more balls, one under each hip, to give yourself a hip massage at the same time. This self-massage often helps to relieve the pain of muscle spasms, strains, or sprains.

Get Out of Bed as Soon as You Can

Try to be up and moving about by the second day. Do not remain in bed longer than three days. By the fourth or fifth day, the pain should have diminished. If it has not, you should see a physician.

You should also see a doctor if back pain follows an injury or is accompanied by fever, vomiting, nausea, sweating, weakness, or abdominal pain; or if you lose bowel or bladder control; or if the pain radiates to the buttocks, thigh, or leg; or if a leg feels numb or tingles; or if the pain is so severe you are unable to move; or if the pain has lasted more than two weeks. With symptoms like these, the pain *could* be due to a wide variety of medical problems, ranging from kidney, prostate, or urinary tract disorders to cystitis, ligament injury, a compression fracture, a hernia, flat feet, unequal leg length, bone spurs, a spinal abnormality, a tumor, nerve root damage, or a problem in the sacroiliac region.

But normally, that is, 95 percent of the time, any lower back pain that comes on suddenly is usually due to muscle spasm resulting from a muscle-injury—and pain can be relieved by the action-steps in Painstopper #50.

If you have read this book so far, you will already know that the underlying cause of most lower back pain is unrelieved emotional stress. After a long, stressful day at the office, and a tiring commute on the freeway, we typically arrive home frustrated and angry. In this stressful mind-set we perceive the world as threatening and hostile. In response to this fear-based emotion, the mind immediately triggers the fight-or-flight response.

Immediately the body goes into an emergency state. Adrenaline is pumped into muscles to charge them with energy. Unless we use this energy for physical exertion, our entire musculature, and our back muscles in particular, become tight with tension. In this taut condition, they are easily torn.

When our abdomen and back muscles are weakened by years of physical inactivity and sedentary living, a simple exertion like leaning forward to raise a window, or bending over to pick up a paint bucket, can tear a rigid back muscle. In self-defense, to prevent further movement and damage, the muscle goes into spasm.

You already know the rest.

■ THE MOST WIDESPREAD CAUSE OF CHRONIC PAIN

Medical records show that lower back pain is the most common and widespread form of chronic pain. Each day, 6.5 million Americans must stay in bed, or miss work, due to crippling pain in the lower back. And each year, 18 million Americans visit the doctor complaining of persistent lower back pain.

Statistics show that once lower back pain occurs, you are 4 times as likely to have it again. After age 45, back pain becomes a recurring problem for one in three Americans. And unless something is done, lower back pain becomes progressively worse and occurs more frequently.

Not surprisingly, back pain relief has become a thriving industry with tens of thousands of back care specialists and practitioners together with dozens of lumbar support devices ranging from kneeling chairs to do-it-yourself traction units, back-oriented chairs and pillows, and car seat inserts. All are fairly expensive, and results are often so disappointing that one back specialist recently estimated that a rolled-up towel could do more to relieve back pain than almost any of these devices.

■ RECOMMENDATIONS FOR BACK PAIN RELIEF

Yoga Beats Medical Science in Relieving Back Pain

Most back specialists or practitioners cannot offer any panacea. Several years ago, a survey of back pain patients by New York market researcher Arthur C. Klein and his science writer wife found that the best and most successful back pain therapists were yoga instructors: 96 percent of their students with lower back pain attained long-term pain relief. Next came physiatrists (medical doctors specializing in musculoskeletal rehabilitation) with a success rate of 86 percent, followed by physical therapists (65 percent), acupuncturists (36 percent), chiropractors (28 percent), orthopedists (26 percent), neurosurgeons (23 percent), internists and family practitioners (20 percent), and neurologists (4 percent).

According to the survey participants, every therapist except the yoga instructors failed to help some patients and made some patients feel worse. The neurologists prescribed more drugs than any other therapists, were ineffective 76 percent of the time, and made 16 percent of their patients feel worse. As a general rule, I might add that, the higher a specialist's fees, the lower the success rate. And while several of these therapies remain controversial for the relief of back pain, specialists in each continue to argue that theirs is the only way to go.

Thanks to the survey, we now know that yoga (muscle stretching, relaxation, and stress management) and physiatry (muscle rehabilitation) are by far the best therapies for long-term relief from lower back pain. With their combined success rate of 91 percent, it is safe to say that, once the possibility of disease or dysfunction has been ruled out, nine out of every ten cases of chronic lower back pain can be completely and permanently eliminated without surgery or drugs.

Don't Take Back Pain Lying Down

Let's assume you have just recovered from your latest flare-up of acute lower back pain. Your doctor has checked you out and given you medical clearance. You can now move normally once more, and you are free of pain. But you are still vulnerable, and you realize that your back could go out again at any time. You also know that each time your back muscles go into spasm, the pain becomes worse and recovery takes longer.

The good news is that you don't *have* to go on suffering and living in fear. By adopting a strategy based on yoga and physiatry you can

1. Rebuild your weak and flabby back and abdomen muscles and increase their flexibility. In this way, good body mechanics is restored, and lower back pain is unable to occur again.
2. Restore your weight to normal through diet and aerobic exercise. This is a necessary step because carrying just 10 pounds of excess weight on the abdomen can exert 50 pounds of resistance whenever you move your back muscles. Most Americans with lower back pain rarely exercise their abdominals, and they gradually acquire a pot belly. Having even a small pot belly frequently leads to one back strain after another. Yet lower back pain is virtually unknown in fit people who exercise regularly.
3. Upgrade your life-style to reduce the psychological stress that is the underlying cause of lower back pain.

Achieve a Lifetime of Freedom From Chronic Back Pain

Providing you're willing to practice behavioral medicine—that is, to use your mind and muscles actively—you clearly and definitely can achieve a lifetime of freedom from chronic lower back pain. All it takes is to adopt and practice the exercises described in the next major section, "The Number One Program for a Pain-Free Back."

You begin with Painstopper #51: Program for a Pain-Free Back—The Warm-up, and then continue on, one by one, with ten simple painstopper exercises. Almost all the exercises are yoga stretches or back-building exercises. Each has been tested and proven in hundreds of professionally supervised programs designed to build healthy backs.

So learn to do as many as you can. And count on doing a total of 15–30 minutes of combined warm-up and back exercises at least 5 times a week or, preferably, once each day.

Practiced regularly, these physical action-steps should prevent the recurrence of most chronic lower back pain. However, they may not entirely overcome the effects of being seriously overweight or severely over-stressed. Thus, for a complete whole-person approach, I recommend that you also adopt the following painstopper strategies described in earlier chapters.

Painstopper #2: Walk Away from Pain
Painstopper #3: The One Diet That Does It All

Later, as your weight becomes normal and your muscles are stronger and more flexible, you can begin to reduce the emotional stress that is the underlying cause of most chronic back pain. To accomplish this, I recommend adopting the following painstopper techniques.

Painstopper #9: Relaxation Training—Nature's Prescription for Pain Relief
Painstopper #21: Keep Pain at Bay with Positive Beliefs

You should also read and absorb all of Chapter 8 (including the Ten Affirmations That May Help Reduce Stress and Relieve Your Chronic Pain). Together, these action-steps form a whole-person approach that has proven highly effective in permanently ending chronic lower back pain.

Take the Load Off Your Back

Emphasis in this chapter is on physical action-steps that are frankly designed to take the load off your back. To remain permanently free of back pain, you must maintain these exercises for at least five days each week or, preferably, every day for the rest of your life. If you do not—if you merely exercise until your pain goes away, and then stop—your chronic back pain will inevitably return. And it will keep on recurring and becoming more painful.

If you think I'm an alarmist, consider what happened to Eric G. Eric is a 45-year-old Colorado businessman whose chronic back pain was due to a mix of unresolved stress, sedentary living, and 30 pounds of excess weight.

After several bouts of acute back pain, each of which kept him in bed for several days, Eric enrolled in a "Healthy Back Program" offered by a local health spa. The spa's program was almost identical to "The Number One Program For a Pain-Free Back" described in the next major section of this chapter.

For as long as he kept up his daily exercises, Eric remained totally free of lower back pain. But Eric soon became complacent. He began to skip exercise sessions and to indulge once more in sweets and high-fat foods.

"I figured my back pain had gone, and it wouldn't come back," he told me. "So I gave up exercising altogether. I began to put on extra inches around the waist, and my weight began to creep back up."

A few weeks after that, Eric stooped over to pick up an empty garbage can. Suddenly, a sharp familiar pain shot through his back. He spent the next three days in bed.

"I was right back where I started," Eric said. "So be sure to tell your readers this. Anytime you allow your abdomen muscles to weaken or relapse, and your weight to rise, your back pain will almost certainly return again."

Fortunately, Eric went right back to his healthful life-style, and once more, his back pain has disappeared.

So which is worse? A few hours of healthful exercise each week (which can also prevent heart disease and cancer) or a week of total disablement that is repeated eight or ten times a year?

So I urge you not to make the same mistake as Eric. Instead, persist and stay with these pain-stopping action-steps for life. As scores of studies and surveys have proved, virtually everyone who faithfully practices our exercise program is rewarded with a strong, supple, and pain-free back.

THE NUMBER ONE PROGRAM FOR A PAIN-FREE BACK

Physical therapists have long known that most victims of chronic lower back pain have ramrod-stiff backs and chronically stiff muscles and joints. Hence the following exercise program was specifically designed to elongate the spine and to develop strength and flexibility in your abdomen, hips, hamstring, and back extensor muscles.

As always, I recommend that you have your doctor's permission before adopting any exercise program. Yoga instructors also caution that most yoga stretches are a mild form of traction and should be avoided by women when more than four months pregnant. Should an exercise seem painful, check that you are doing it correctly. If pain persists, cease doing that exercise. No exercise should ever hurt your back. If it does, or if you experience bruises or swelling, stop exercising. On the other hand, don't be put off by a little muscle stiffness or minor muscle ache.

When doing stretches, stretch to the point of feeling minor pain. Then stop, back off slightly, and hold. Also, always exhale while performing the most strenuous part of an exercise.

Some of these exercises may not only prevent lower back pain but help to relieve existing pain. After an attack of acute lower back pain, you can usually begin doing some of the stretching exercises to help relieve the remaining pain provided that it feels comfortable to do so.

Remember, you should do 15–30 minutes of combined warm-up and back exercises on at least five days each week or, preferably, once every day.

PAINSTOPPER #51:
Program for a Pain-Free Back—The Warm-up

Before commencing any strength-building or stretching exercise, we must first warm up by walking or bicycling briskly for at least 5 minutes. Brisk aerobic exercise like this pumps oxygen and nutrients to joints and muscles throughout the body, making them flexible, and strengthens the buttocks, legs, back, and abdominals.

The benefits of aerobic exercise are so numerous that almost all back clinics use walking as the core of their rehabilitation program. For proof, a recent study of 1,652 firefighters revealed that those who did the most aerobic exercise had the best cardiovascular fitness and they experienced only 10 percent of the incapacitating back injuries that afflicted those who did the least aerobic exercise. The study was one of many to demonstrate that lower back pain is almost always the result of sedentary living, and it will continue for as long as a person remains physically inactive and overweight.

So begin by taking an easy walk for just a few minutes. Try to walk tall and relaxed and keep the abdomen as flat as you can to maintain a slight pelvic tilt. There's no upper limit on how far or how fast you can walk to warm up. You can read more about the benefits of walking in Painstopper #2.

If you aren't able to walk or pedal a stationary bicycle, consider walking back and forth immersed to the waist in a fairly warm swimming pool. The water will both support you and provide resistance to exercise against. Avoid a cold pool, however, as you will not warm up. If you simply cannot exercise aerobically, soak in a warm tub for up to 10 minutes before commencing the exercises that follow.

As soon as you have warmed up, begin to do the exercises described in the following 11 painstoppers.

PAINSTOPPER #52:
Program for a Pain-Free Back—The Pelvic Tilt

The pelvic tilt is a magnificent exercise for strengthening the abdominals while stretching the back muscles at the same time.

- *Step 1:* Lie on your back on a rug on the floor. Raise your knees and draw your heels in close to your buttocks. Keep your feet flat on the floor throughout the exercise.

- *Step 2:* Take a deep inhalation. As you slowly exhale,

  Press the lower back flat against the floor.

  Squeeze the buttocks tightly together.

  Suck the abdomen in toward the spine.

  All three steps should be done simultaneously. This will tilt the top of the pelvis forward and down. Hold this pelvic tilt position during the 6–8 seconds it takes to complete a slow exhalation.

- *Step 3:* As you inhale,

  Relax the abdomen.

  Arch the lower back up off the floor so that the weight is on the buttocks.

  Fill the belly with air.

All three steps should be done simultaneously and held for the 6–8 seconds it takes for a slow, deep inhalation.

- *Step 4:* Repeat the exhale-inhale cycle twice more. Then continue on with Painstopper #53.

PAINSTOPPER #53:
Program for a Pain-Free Back—The Crunch-up

Because full sit-ups mainly strengthen the hip flexor muscles, modern physical therapists recommend the crunch-up as a better way to strengthen the abdominal muscles. Additionally, doing crunch-ups strengthens the lower back while also getting you into the pelvic tilt position.

- *Step 1:* Lie on your back on a rug on the floor. Raise your knees and keep your feet flat on the floor throughout this exercise.

- *Step 2:* Exhale as you crunch up and inhale as you relax back down to the floor. Place the hands on the chest with arms crossed. Slowly tuck in your chin and curl your head and neck up until your shoulders are off the floor. Endeavor to move your forehead toward your knees. Move slowly and deliberately to avoid any bouncing.

- *Step 3:* Relax slowly back down to the floor. Then repeat the exercise 9 more times or until you are mildly fatigued. Within a month, most people can do 20 repetitions.

  As your abdominal muscles gain strength, twist slowly as you crunch-up and try to touch one knee with the opposite elbow. Change sides at each crunch-up. This variation will strengthen the abdominal side muscles.

Then continue on with Painstopper #54.

PAINSTOPPER #54:
Program for a Pain-Free Back—The Hamstring Stretch

This is one of several variations of the hamstring stretch. It is designed to stretch the hamstring muscles at the back of the thighs, and you will undoubtedly feel a mild stretch behind your knees.

- *Step 1:* Sit on a mat on the floor with your legs extended straight out and together. Breathe normally throughout this exercise and do not hold the breath.

- *Step 2:* Bend forward and reach out with your hands to grasp the toes on each foot. Keep the knees straight and flat on the floor. If you cannot reach this far, grasp your ankles or calves. Bend over and reach as far as you can. Hold this position for 10 seconds. Then release and straighten back up. Repeat two more times.

- *Step 3:* As you become more limber, try this variation. Sit on the floor with legs extended. Bend one knee and draw in the foot until the heel is as close to your crotch as you can bring it. The outer side of your foot should be on the floor with the sole of your foot against your other thigh. Now lower the knee as close to the floor as you can.

  Then bend down and reach forward with both hands to grasp the toes of the extended leg. Hold this position for 10 seconds, and release. Repeat with the other leg. Then repeat the entire exercise twice more.

Continue on with Painstopper #55.

PAINSTOPPER #55:
Program for a Pain-Free Back—The Knee-to-Chest Curl

Step 1: Lie on your back on a rug on the floor with knees raised and feet about 12 inches apart.

- *Step 2:* Raise one knee and pull it into your chest with clasped hands. Bounce this knee into your chest 20 – 40 times. Then release and repeat with the other knee.

- *Step 3:* Raise both knees together and pull into your chest with clasped hands. Bounce your knees into your chest 20 – 40 times. Relax and lower your legs to the floor. Repeat 2 more times.

- *Step 4:* Raise both knees together and pull into your chest with clasped hands. Pull in your knees as close to your chest as you can. Hold this position. As you exhale, raise head, neck, and shoulders off the floor in the crunch-up position (see Painstopper #53). Hold 6–8 seconds or until you begin to inhale. Repeat this step a total of 5 times.

Continue on with Painstopper #56.

PAINSTOPPER #56:
Program for a Pain-Free Back—The Swayback Spine Flexor

This splendid spine-flexing exercise will swiftly remove all stiffness from the spine while also stretching both back and abdomen muscles.

- *Step 1:* Go down on hands and knees on a rug on the floor so that your back is parallel to the floor.

- *Step 2:* Take a deep breath. Then, as you exhale, simultaneously

Arch your spine as high as you can like an angry cat.
Drop your head and neck as low as you can and tuck in your chin.
Suck in your abdomen toward your spine.

Hold these combined positions throughout the exhalation. Ideally, that could be 5–8 seconds.

- *Step 3:* Immediately when you begin to inhale, reverse the stance and behave like a swayback horse carrying a 500-pound load:

Flex your spine to give it a real caved-in hollow.

Relax the abdomen and fill the belly with air.

Raise chin, head, and neck as high as possible and look up as high as you can.

Hold these combined positions throughout the inhalation. Ideally, that could be 5–8 seconds.

- *Step 4:* Repeat the entire exercise up to 10 times in rhythm with your breathing. Avoid moving fast as it creates bounce and momentum.

Continue on with Painstopper #57.

PAINSTOPPER #57:
Program for a Pain-Free Back—Leg Lowering

For anyone with a back problem, leg-lowering strengthens the abdominal muscles and stretches the back just as effectively as leg-raising does and with minimal risk of straining the back.

- *Step 1:* Lie flat on your back on a rug on the floor with arms on the floor at your sides. Keep your legs straight, and breathe normally, throughout the exercise.

- *Step 2:* Raise one leg slowly as high as you can and hold it there. Next, slowly raise the other leg to the same height. Keep the legs together now. You can take 3 – 4 seconds to raise each leg.

- *Step 3:* Lower both legs together back to the floor as slowly as you can. You can take as long as you like—the slower you go, the greater the benefit.

- *Step 4:* All movements should be slow and deliberate. Repeat the entire exercise at least three times, or for as many times as you like.

Continue on with Painstopper #58.

PAINSTOPPER #58:
Program for a Pain-Free Back—The Easy Bridge Pose

This easy yoga posture strengthens the back muscles while increasing spinal flexibility.

- *Step 1:* Lie on your back on a rug on the floor with knees raised and feet flat on the floor. Your heels should be about 6 inches from your buttocks.

- *Step 2:* Keeping your shoulders on the floor, raise your buttocks as high off the floor as you can.

- *Step 3:* Hold 6 seconds, or longer, and lower your buttocks back to the floor. Repeat 5–6 times, more if you like.

Continue on with Painstopper #59.

PAINSTOPPER #59:
Program for a Pain-Free Back—The Cobra Pose

After flexing backward in this popular yoga posture, your spine should feel almost as flexible as a cobra's. As you arch the spine back, the cobra pose also gives a good stretch to the abdomen and quadricep muscles.

- *Step 1:* Lay on a rug on the floor, face down and on your stomach, with legs straight and together. Place your hands palms down on the rug, one beneath each shoulder.

- *Step 2:* Using the back muscles, raise your head and chest off the floor as high as you can; then use the arms to continue to raise the chest and shoulders as high as possible. After a few attempts, most people can straighten their arms. The spine is now arched back. Raise your chin and look up as high as you can. Keep the pelvis and abdomen on the floor.

  Hold for 10 seconds and slowly lower back to the floor.

- *Step 3:* As you progress, add this variation. While holding the cobra pose, raise your lower legs from the knee and bring your heels as close to your buttocks as you can. Hold for 10 seconds and return to the basic cobra pose.

As you progress, you can hold the cobra and the bent-knee positions for longer periods. The longer you hold, the more flexible your back will become.

Continue on with Painstopper #60.

PAINSTOPPER #60:
Program for a Pain-Free Back—The Lateral Stretch

This exercise gives a sideways stretch to the entire spine while strengthening both the abdominal and back muscles.

- *Step 1:* Stand erect with legs spread wide apart and feet flat on the floor. Clasp your hands together and place them on top of your head.

- *Step 2:* Inhale. Then as you exhale, bend the trunk sideways and down as far as you can to the right. Avoid bending or twisting forward.

- *Step 3:* As you inhale, return to the upright position. Without stopping, begin to exhale and continue to bend as far as you can to the left.

- *Step 4:* Without stopping, begin to inhale and return to the upright position. Begin to exhale and continue on to bend as far as you can to the right.

   Without stopping, keep up the side-to-side bending motion in rhythm with your breath. Try to move deliberately without bouncing or using momentum. Repeat 5 times each way, or as many times as you like.

   Continue on with Painstopper #61.

PAINSTOPPER #61:
Program for a Pain-Free Back—The Spinal Extension

By stretching the lumbar extensor muscles in the lower back, this exercise not only prevents lower back pain but may also relieve it.

- *Step 1:* Lie face down on a rug on the floor. Clench the fists loosely and place them, knuckles down, on the rug under each of your hips.

- *Step 2:* Keeping the right leg straight, raise it as high in the air as you can. Hold it there 6 seconds, and slowly lower. Repeat with the left leg. Continue to alternate 10 times with each leg. As you progress, hold each leg as high as you can for a longer period. It may help to place a pillow under the pelvis.

- *Step 3:* Once you can do step 2, begin to raise both legs together. Keep them straight and raise them as high as you can. Hold for 6 seconds, and slowly lower. As you progress, hold your legs as high as you can for a longer period. You can continue to keep the pillow under the pelvis.

- *Step 4:* Remove the pillow from under the pelvis. Remove the arms from under the hips and place them on the floor reaching straight out overhead. Now, keeping both arms and legs straight, simultaneously raise both off the floor. Raise the head off the floor and look up at the arms. Only the abdomen remains fully on the floor. Hold for 6 seconds and slowly lower back to the floor. As you progress, you can hold this posture—actually the yoga "canoe" pose—for an increasingly longer period.

PAINSTOPPER #62:
Seven Steps to Safeguard Yourself from Lower Back Pain

Most cases of lower back pain are triggered by seven common life-style causes. Here's how you can prevent them from causing pain for you.

- *Step 1:* Use correct body mechanics when lifting. Lift with your arm and leg muscles, not your back. Keep your back straight when lifting and your pelvis tucked in. Bend at the hips and knees and lift by straightening your knees and raising your arms. Never hunch over a weight to lift it or arch, curve, or twist your back as you lift. Take a deep breath before lifting and exert yourself as you exhale. Never lift a weight higher than your waist. If you must lift heavy weights, wear a nylon lifting belt—a stiff belt 4–5 inches wide available at fitness and weight-lifting stores—that supports and stabilizes the abdomen and lower back.

- *Step 2:* Sleep on a firm mattress. If your back aches when you wake up, your mattress may be too soft. Try sleeping on the floor on three blankets, each folded in two. If you wake up for several mornings without an ache, your mattress may need firming up. To stiffen it, insert a piece of 3/4-inch plywood beneath your mattress.

- *Step 3:* Sleep correctly. If backache appears after sleeping, try sleeping on your side with hips and knees flexed in the fetal position. Place a thin pillow between the knees to improve circulation. If you sleep on your back, place a thick pillow under your knees to keep your spine straight. Avoid sleeping on your stomach. However you sleep, use a firm pillow.

- *Step 4:* Sit correctly. Never slouch while sitting and try to avoid sitting in overstuffed chairs. Just as bad are low, deep-cushioned chairs or couches into which you sink down. Try to always sit in a chair with a firm back. Sit upright with your spine as straight as possible. Keep your back flattened against the chair and your pelvis tilted back. This advice also applies while driving. Many people prefer to place a pillow behind their back while driving to help keep the spine straight.

- *Step 5:* Keep moving. Never stand or sit in one position for longer than 30 minutes without getting up and moving around. If you must stand for a long period, elevate one foot at a time by placing it on a low stool. Whenever possible, rise up and down on the toes and flex the calves to improve circulation. While on the telephone, try to walk around. Take a few steps whenever you can. Better, take a short walk every half hour and flex every muscle in your arms, legs, torso, shoulders, neck, and hips. Try to avoid driving or riding in a car for long periods.

- *Step 6:* Avoid these exercises. Avoid doing full sit-ups or full leg raises when exercising and also avoid the breast or butterfly strokes while swimming. Also *never* wear high heels.

- *Step 7:* Stand tall. Stand or walk tall and erect with your back straight and pelvis slightly tucked in. Imagine that your entire body is suspended from a hook in the top of your head and you are hanging loose and relaxed with your spine perpendicular. Try to lead off all movements with your head so that your spine and the rest of your body follows.

As any back specialist will tell you, it's many times easier to *prevent* lower back pain than it is to try and relieve it after it happens.

Chapter 12

TAKE THE OFFENSIVE AGAINST PAIN

With This Arsenal of Physical Therapies for Ending the Pain of Specific Ailments

This chapter describes more physical action-steps for relieving the pain of specific conditions other than arthritis, headaches, and lower back pain. If you don't find anything listed for your particular type of pain, it may be because no really effective way exists of relieving that pain by any Class III action-step.

For instance, you won't find anything in this chapter for relieving pain due to cancer, AIDS, burns, fractures, injuries, or surgery. That's because no Class III painstopper action-steps exist for easing the pain of these conditions.

Instead, I recommend using a combination of Class I and Class II painstoppers. As you may recall, Class I painstoppers are physical action-steps that are effective for every kind of pain, while Class II painstoppers are mental action-steps that are also effective for every kind of pain. All Class I painstoppers are listed in Chapter 4, and all Class II painstoppers are described in Chapters 5 through 8.

By combining one or more Class I painstoppers with one or more Class II painstoppers, you can still put together a highly effective whole-person program for relieving almost any pain.

Meanwhile, here is the pick of the best and most successful physical therapies for relieving the pain of specific ailments and conditions.

ABDOMINAL PAINS

Approximately one American in two has a recurrent ailment that causes pain and discomfort in the gastrointestinal tract. Not all abdominal pain lends itself to natural treatment. New drugs have replaced surgery as a cure for ulcers, and ulcers have become quite rare, especially in older people.

Nonetheless, conditions like diverticulosis, irritable bowel syndrome, and gallbladder problems still abound and continue to make life miserable for millions of Americans. Painstopper techniques that may help to relieve several types of common abdominal pain are described here.

PAINSTOPPER #63:
Self-help for Diverticulitis Pain

Persistent cramps, bloating, nausea, and mild to severe pain in the lower left abdomen may be symptoms of diverticulitis or inflammation of the lining of the lower colon. The pain is usually caused by a diet that is deficient in fiber. When food residues lack sufficient fiber, they clog the tiny pouches that line the colon wall, causing them to bulge out and become inflamed. It is this inflammation that is responsible for the pain of diverticulitis.

Over half of all Americans eat a diet that is low in fiber, and the majority suffer from diverticulosis, a condition in which their colon wall could become inflamed at any time. Although most cases of diverticulitis are mild enough to turn around by natural means, more advanced cases can be quite serious and may call for bed rest and antibiotics. Anyone with diverticulosis symptoms should consult a physician as soon as convenient.

However, if your doctor gives you a medical go-ahead, you can usually phase out your diverticulitis pain within 7–14 days, and you need never experience it again.

The solution is to switch to a high-fiber diet of plant-based foods such as fruits, vegetables, legumes, whole grains, seeds, and nuts. The change-over should be made gradually to avoid creating gas or flatulence.

With your doctor's cooperation and approval, I recommend adopting Painstopper #3: The One Diet That Does it All. Keep cutting down on all foods that are low in fiber. Low-fiber foods include all flesh foods; eggs; dairy foods (including cheese, sour cream, and ice cream); most fried foods; fats, oils, and margarine; and all refined flours and sweeteners. Replace these low-residue foods with increasing amounts of vegetables, fruits, legumes, and whole grains plus some sunflower seeds and a few nuts each day.

Besides helping to phase out diverticulitis pain, these same high-fiber foods will significantly reduce your risk of ever getting heart disease, stroke, cancer, diabetes, or any other types of abdominal pain.

By making Painstopper #3 a permanent part of your life-style, you are also very unlikely to ever experience diverticulitis pain in the first place.

PAINSTOPPER #64:
Self-help for Irritable Bowel Syndrome

Persistent pain in the abdomen with bloating, cramps, diarrhea, and constipation sounds a lot like the symptoms of diverticulitis. But if you're under age 40, and a woman — or a man who is prone to stress — your problem may be irritable bowel syndrome instead. Women who are highly educated and perfectionists seem to get irritable bowel syndrome most often.

As this was written, irritable bowel syndrome could not be diagnosed by lab tests or by a physical exam. Nonetheless, you should have a medical check-up to eliminate the possibility of a more life-threatening condition. Your physician may prescribe antispasmodic or antidiarrheal drugs.

But you can usually say goodbye to irritable bowel syndrome in just a short time by combining four of our painstopper techniques to form an all-natural, whole-person, pain-healing program.

With your doctor's approval, you should lose no time in adopting and practicing

Painstopper #2: Walk Away from Pain

Painstopper #3: The One Diet That Does it All

Painstopper #9: Relaxation Training

Painstopper #11: Biofeedback Training

Combining diet with exercise and relaxation, these painstopper action-steps should end the pain and discomfort of irritable bowel syndrome in just a short time.

PAINSTOPPER #65:
Natural Ways to Relieve Gallbladder Pain

A sudden intense pain on the right side of the abdomen, that intensifies and then lasts several hours before fading, may well be due to a gallbladder problem. If the pain radiates into, or below, the right shoulder blade, it may indicate a stone impacted in the bile duct. Gallbladder pain may also be accompanied by cold, fever, nausea, sweating, chills, or a yellow skin color (jaundice). After a few hours, the pain fades away but returns again at intervals.

The gallbladder is a pouch tucked in the lobes of the liver that collects bile and conveys it to the small intestine. Through years of eating foods high in fat and cholesterol, stones of cholesterol may form and block the duct. This prevents bile from being ejected into the small intestine where it is needed to digest fat. Dietary fat then passes undigested through the intestines, imparting a clay color to stools.

- *Step 1:* To relieve the pain, take a long, hot soak in a tub bath. Since heat dilates and relaxes all blood vessels and body parts, it may also help in passing a gallstone.

- *Step 2:* Next, apply contrasting heat and cold. Place a hot pack on the painful area of the abdomen at the same time as you place a cold pack on the small of the back. Remove the cold pack as soon as the back feels numb and remove the hot pack after 20 – 30 minutes.

- *Step 3:* Begin immediately to change over to a diet high in fiber and very low in fat (see Painstopper #3 for details).

- *Step 4:* Break up each normal-size meal into three minimeals, making a total of nine small meals. Eat each minimeal at equally spaced intervals throughout the day.

Every year, over 500,000 Americans have gallbladder surgery, and the majority are overweight people who eat a high-fat diet, people over 60, and young Native American women.

Taken in time, the preceding action-steps may save you from surgery while the gallbladder pain may gradually disappear. Nonetheless, anyone with gallbladder pain is urged to see a doctor without delay. If an operation is recommended, obtain an unbiased second opinion before consenting.

FIBROSITIS PAIN

This arthritic dysfunction, also known as fibromyalgia or fibromyositis, affects over 7 million Americans, mostly women aged 20 – 55. The pain may last from four days to four months or longer but eventually disappears. Longer-lasting fibrositis is often due to unresolved emotional stress that creates tension deep within muscles. Painful trigger points then develop in these muscles, causing muscle tenderness and pain to appear, primarily in the neck, hip, knee, lower back, or elbow. Any fibrositis symptoms should be checked out by a physician to eliminate the possibility of a more serious problem and to establish that your pain is really caused by the fibrositis.

Assuming you are given medical clearance, fibrositis often responds well to a whole-person approach based on a combination of

Painstopper #2: Walk Away from Pain

Painstopper #9: Relaxation Training—Nature's Prescription for Pain
　　　　　　　　Relief

Painstopper #11: Biofeedback Training—Mind over Pain

Painstopper #21: Keep Pain at Bay with Positive Beliefs

You should also be certain to obtain adequate sleep. The pain and muscle tenderness caused by fibrositis may also respond well to gentle muscle stretching. Low back pain is one of the most common forms of fibrositis pain. Painstopper #66 describes a simple stretching technique for relieving it.

PAINSTOPPER #66:
Relieving Low Back Pain Due to Fibrositis

Fibrositis trigger points in muscles deep within the spine and ribs frequently cause severe low back pain. This pain can usually be relieved by a simple "ear-to-knee" stretch.

- *Step 1:* Sit on an upright chair with knees wide apart. Bend forward and down so that your head drops between your knees. Keeping your arms outside your knees, clasp your right ankle with your right hand and your left ankle with your left hand. Then continue to bend the torso down as far as you can.

- *Step 2:* Gently bend the trunk to the right as far as you can without discomfort, and stretch until your right ear touches your right knee.

- *Step 3:* As you hold the position you reached in step 2, turn your head gently as far to the right as you can. Then raise your left arm until your elbow comes as close as possible to your left ear. Hold this position for 15 seconds, then release.

- *Step 4:* Repeat on the other side by touching the left ear to the left knee and raising the right arm up to cover your right ear.

ANGINA, CLAUDICATION, AND HEARTBURN PAIN

For months, Jerry R. had experienced a dull ache in his chest and left arm whenever he did any physical exertion. Then one afternoon, while walking on the golf course, he felt a crushing pain in his chest.

Thoroughly frightened, Jerry dropped to the ground. Sweat poured from his brow. The heavy squeezing sensation in his chest radiated into his left arm and shoulder. Jerry felt as though a tight band was squeezing the life out of his chest.

The pain lasted only a few minutes and then began to subside. Jerry lay exhausted, sucking in huge gulps of air. He completed the trip to the clubhouse in a golf cart.

Whenever he exerted himself after that, the same oppressive pain returned. Jerry called his internist for an appointment.

The very next day, after taking a series of tests, Jerry sat facing his internist in the doctor's office.

"No, you didn't have a heart attack," his doctor reassured him. "Your pain is due to stable angina, meaning that your coronary arteries are so blocked with cholesterol plaque that your heart muscle lacks the oxygen it needs to pump blood throughout your body."

The doctor handed Jerry several small bottles of nitroglycerine pills with instructions to dissolve one under his tongue if the pain came back. The doctor also told Jerry that anyone with angina was in constant danger of having a heart attack and that he would later prescribe a maintenance drug to prevent the angina from recurring. Jerry would have to take this drug for the rest of his life.

Jerry R. Discovers the Benefits of Becoming a Medically Informed Layperson

Jerry spent the next five evenings poring over medical books and journals at the public library. Angina pain, he learned, is caused when the heart muscle is deprived of oxygen. This can occur in one of two ways.

Stable angina occurs when cholesterol deposits occlude a coronary artery, preventing blood from reaching the heart muscle. Angina pain then occurs with exertion. *Mixed* angina occurs when the muscles that surround each artery go into spasm, constricting the coronary arteries, and also preventing blood from reaching the heart muscle. Pain may then occur at any time, whether at rest or when beginning to exercise. However, mixed angina pain seldom occurs once exercise is in progress.

At first, Jerry feared that open heart surgery might eventually be needed to end his angina pain. But as he read more recent medical literature, he learned that angina pain can often be stopped without either surgery or drugs.

Until recent years, the only medically accepted remedy for angina was lifelong medication often supplemented by major surgery. Even then, unless key life-style changes are made to lower dietary fat and increase exercise, the coronary arteries may again become clogged in just a few years.

Right then, Jerry realized that mainstream medicine may not have the real answer to angina pain. Instead of dealing with the cause, drugs and surgery merely treat the symptoms of heart disease.

His conclusion was prompted by learning that since 1977, behavioral medicine has been successfully used to reverse tens of thousands of cases of angina pain without surgery or drugs. In 1989, Dean Ornish scientifically proved that the pain of stable angina could be permanently relieved through a combination of exercise, a very low-fat diet, and stress management.

Bypass operations continue to be done because millions of Americans are unwilling to use their minds and muscles to help themselves beat angina pain. In stark contrast, literally hundreds of cardiac rehabilitation centers have opened across the country. These centers use behavioral medicine to permanently end the pain of angina (and, in many cases, the even worse pain of intermittent claudication—an intense pain in the legs that occurs when walking in people whose arteries are blocked with cholesterol plaque).

Relieving Angina Pain with Behavioral Medicine

As he grasped these facts, Jerry decided to enroll at a nearby cardiac rehabilitation clinic. After his angina was medically evaluated, Jerry was put on a program that is virtually identical to a combination of our Painstoppers #2, #3, #9, and #21. All participants in the program also had to stop smoking.

Under medical supervision, Jerry immediately commenced a program of gradually increasing daily walking exercise coupled with a very low-fat diet. He also learned to relax and to let go of stress.

Results were dramatic.

Without ever being put on any kind of drug or medication, Jerry's angina pains began to diminish steadily. A final mild attack occurred during his fourth week on the program. Since then, he has not experienced any pain. The reason is that he briskly walks 3 miles every day, and he intends to stay with his low-fat diet for the rest of his life.

At our last contact, Jerry had been free of angina for nearly two years. He had never felt better, and he had no intention of ever going back to his former sedentary life-style and high-fat diet—the same health-destroying habits that caused his angina in the first place.

A Word of Caution

Any type of angina or claudication is a form of heart disease. So before beginning any program to relieve stable or mixed angina, or claudication, you absolutely *must* have your pain medically examined and diagnosed.

And since any form of heart disease involves the possibility of a heart attack, you *must* have your doctor's full and complete permission, approval, and cooperation before using any of our painstoppers to phase out angina or claudication. If your doctor medicalizes everything and tends to see solutions only in terms of medical treatment, consider getting a second opinion from a more holistically oriented physician, preferably one who is familiar with behavioral medicine.

If at this time you are free of heart disease but wish to use our painstoppers to prevent heart disease or angina from ever occurring, your doctor's approval is all you need to go ahead and use them.

Important Note: These painstoppers may not work if you are still smoking.

PAINSTOPPER #67:
The Ultimate Way to Permanently End the Pain of Stable Angina

The modern way to phase out chest pain due to stable angina is to begin using the following two painstoppers, each described earlier in this book.

Painstopper #2: Walk Away from Pain
Painstopper #3: The One Diet That Does it All

From the original Pritikin Program that first reversed heart disease naturally in 1977 to the most recent regimes to emerge from the nation's top university medical centers, all are virtually identical with our Painstoppers #2 and #3. To complete a whole-person approach, you merely need to add two other Painstoppers.

Painstopper #9: Relaxation Training—Nature's Prescription for Pain Relief
Painstopper #21: Keep Pain at Bay with Positive Beliefs

You should also read all of Chapter 8, including the Ten Affirmations That May Help Reduce Stress and Relieve Your Chronic Pain.

I'm not claiming that these painstoppers will ream out your arteries and restore them like new. But results from several recent exercise-and-diet studies indicate that stable angina pain frequently diminishes, or even disappears, a few weeks into the program. Meanwhile, slowly but inexorably, occluded coronary arteries may begin to gradually open up and allow more blood to reach the heart.

PAINSTOPPER #68:

A Common Nutrient That May Prevent the Pain of Mixed Angina

The pain of mixed angina is similar in every way to that of stable angina. But mixed angina occurs when the smooth muscles surrounding the coronary arteries constrict and clamp down, holding these blood vessels shut in a viselike grip. The most common causes of coronary artery spasm are severe emotional stress or a deficiency of the mineral magnesium.

Although it doesn't work for everyone, thousands of Americans have ended the pain of mixed angina by taking up to 400 mg of supplemental magnesium every day. Several types of magnesium supplements are available at health food stores and at many drugstores and supermarkets. Those that include calcium are probably the best for relieving mixed angina.

Generally, it takes a month or so after the supplementation begins to notice a decrease in the frequency and intensity of pain due to spasm in the coronary arteries.

To ensure success, you should strictly avoid caffeinated sodas, alcohol, or certain medications for which artery spasm is an adverse side effect. Some people may also have to avoid caffeine altogether.

I might mention also that a combination of magnesium and calcium supplements has also helped some people to end skipped heartbeats. You can increase your uptake of magnesium by eating more avocados, nuts, peas, and beans.

Even if magnesium is key to ending your mixed angina, I also urge you to make the health-building steps in Painstoppers #2, #3, #9, #11, and #21 a permanent part of your life-style. Stress is also a major cause of mixed angina and the action-steps in these painstoppers form a powerful combination for beating stress.

PAINSTOPPER #69:
Lessening the Pain of Intermittent Claudication

Intermittent claudication is an intense pain in the legs that occurs when walking. It is due to blockage of arteries in the legs by cholesterol plaque and calcium deposits. Like angina, claudication pain can be gradually reduced, or even ended entirely, by using the principles of behavioral medicine.

Just recently, for example, researchers at the Mayo Clinic discovered that the following behavioral medicine action-steps improved circulation in the legs and allowed patients with claudication to walk considerably further without pain. The steps were

- *Step 1:* Walk until the pain forces you to stop.

- *Step 2:* Rest until the pain disappears.

- *Step 3:* Walk again until the pain stops you once more.

- *Step 4:* Keep on repeating steps 1 through 3.

- *Step 5: Immediately and right now,* eliminate virtually all sources of fat, oils, or fried food in the diet together with most flesh and dairy foods (except plain nonfat yogurt, skim milk, and egg whites). Instead, eat a high-fiber diet of plant-based foods. Our Painstopper #3: The One Diet That Does it All describes in detail a diet that is almost identical to that recommended by the Mayo Clinic researchers.

- *Step 6:* Since people with intermittent claudication often suffer from cold feet, in anything but the warmest weather, wear thick wool socks to keep your feet warm. Otherwise, people with this condition may burn their feet while attempting to warm them.

Also, it wouldn't hurt to read and practice the advice in Painstoppers #2, #9, #11, and #21.

Gradually, as circulation improves, more oxygen is able to reach cells throughout the legs, reducing the pain of intermittent claudication and lessening the risk of gangrene or a blood clot.

PAINSTOPPER #70:
Relieving Heartburn Pain Naturally

While heartburn hardly ranks as a major source of chronic pain, it is frequently mistaken for angina or a heart attack. Heartburn typically appears as a burning sensation of fullness or pressure under the breastbone. Genuine heartburn can usually be relieved by taking an antacid. If, despite taking an antacid, the pain and fullness persist, and are accompanied by nausea, sweating, shortness of breath, dizziness, a feeling of fright or panic, or chest pain radiating into the arms, jaw, or back, you *could* be experiencing a heart attack. If you never have had this type of pain before, you should call 911 and request medical help.

Assuming you have ordinary or garden-type heartburn, however, your pain is being caused by stomach acid washing up into the esophagus and burning tissue in the throat. If natural remedies or antacids do not relieve the pain in a week, you should still consult a doctor. Unrelieved heartburn may lead to an ulcer or damage the esophagus.

Lying down usually worsens heartburn pain. Instead, try these home remedies, one by one.

1. Eat a tablespoon of rice pudding.
2. Drink a small cupful of milk.
3. Swallow two capsules of powdered ginger root (available in health food stores) and take up to two more if needed.
4. Stop smoking and drinking alcohol.
5. Avoid chocolate, coffee (including decaffeinated), peppermint, fried or fatty foods, baking soda, citrus, onions, cabbage, chili, and tomatoes.
6. Eat smaller and more frequent meals and avoid eating anything at least 3 hours before bedtime.
7. Raise the head of your bed 6–8 inches. Raising your head and shoulders up on pillows may not work. You may have to raise your mattress or the entire head of the bed. This is one of the best remedies, because it prevents acid flowing into the esophagus.
8. Avoid bending over to pick something up. Squat and bend your knees instead.

9. Wear suspenders instead of a belt and avoid wearing tight clothes.

10. Lose some weight.

Using one or more of these natural pain relievers is almost always preferable to depending on antacids or prescription medication.

KNEE PAIN

Most knee pain can be alleviated, or even eliminated, by natural means. For starters, any persistent knee pain should be examined and diagnosed by an orthopedist or sports medicine specialist, or by a general practitioner if no specialist is available. Most knee pain is due to damage to either a ligament or to cartilage. Any ligament injury should be left entirely in the hands of an orthopedist. But knee pain due to cartilage damage often responds well to exercises designed to rehabilitate the knee. As I've emphasized throughout this book, your physician's approval is essential before you begin using any of the action-steps in this section on knee pain.

Cartilage is a flexible, shock-absorbing tissue on which the kneecap and knee joint glide. Pain occurs when cartilage becomes roughened, worn, pitted, or eroded by overuse or underuse or by injury. Admittedly, it is difficult to restore cartilage damage without surgery.

Yet the real underlying cause of cartilage damage is loss of strength and flexibility in the muscles of the thigh. These muscles, specifically the quadriceps on the front of the thigh, and the hamstrings on the back of the thigh, support the knee and cushion the joint from shock. For as long as these muscles stay weak, cartilage in the knee joint may continue to degenerate. Weak thigh muscles also allow the kneecap to glide out of its proper track and to roughen cartilage behind the kneecap.

Through strengthening the thigh muscles and keeping them flexible, we can prevent further cartilage damage, and we can usually lessen several types of cartilage-caused knee pain, or even clear up the pain altogether. Strengthening the thigh muscles can also postpone onset of osteoarthritis or other forms of knee damage.

The specific action-steps to use depend on where the knee pain is located.

■ **PAIN ON THE OUTSIDE OF THE KNEE**

Pain in this location is often due to a tight iliotibial band, a band of tissue that reaches from hip to knee on the outside of the thigh.

PAINSTOPPER #71:
Relieving Knee Pain Caused by a Tight Iliotibial Band

This type of knee pain may often be relieved by stretching the iliotibial band.

- *Step 1:* Stand sideways about 10 inches from a wall with your painful knee next to the wall.

- *Step 2:* Hold on to the wall for support. Cross the leg with the painful knee behind the other knee. Keep the painful knee straight.

- *Step 3:* Bend the front knee and allow the hip of the painful leg to lean in and touch the wall. Keep the painful leg straight at all times.

- *Step 4:* With the hip of the painful leg against the wall, lean inward and give a thorough stretch to the painful-leg knee. You may want to move slightly farther from the wall to provide a really good stretch. Hold the stretch for 10 seconds; then relax.

    Repeat this stretch 9 more times.

If after a few days, this stretch fails to relieve the pain, the problem may be due to excessive pronation (the inward rolling of the foot when walking). Pronation can often be relieved with an inexpensive over-the-counter orthotic (available in drugstores) or, failing that, with a prescription orthotic.

■ **PAIN UNDER THE KNEECAP**

Pain under the kneecap is often due to chondromalacia, a condition in which weak quadricep (and hamstring) muscles create an imbalance that causes the kneecap to track out of its groove. This inappropriate tracking leads to wear, softening, pitting, and roughening of the cartilage behind the kneecap.

The pain is a dull ache under the kneecap that frequently occurs when descending stairs or a hill or after sitting. The knee may also crack when bending. The immediate cause is weak quadricep muscles that throw the kneecap off center. And the best solution is to strengthen the quadriceps with exercise.

PAINSTOPPER #72:
Relieving Knee Pain Due to Chondromalacia

Never do any of the following exercises to the point of pain. If your knee begins to hurt during these exercises, reduce the weight and cut down on the number of repetitions.

- *Step 1:* Cut back on exercise (walking, running, or bicycling) to where the pain disappears. Never squat or do deep knee bends.

- *Step 2:* Always warm up and stretch before exercising and cool down and stretch after exercising.

  To warm up, take a brief 3 to 4 minute walk, starting at an easy pace and gradually increasing speed.

  To stretch your hamstring muscles, sit on the floor with your legs straight out in front of you. Lean forward and grasp your big toes. If you cannot reach this far, bend forward and reach out as far as you can and grasp the farthest point on your legs that you *can* reach. Hold this stretch for a full minute. Try to increase the stretch until you reach your toes.

  To stretch your quadricep muscles, lie on a rug on the floor on your left side. Bend your right knee and raise your right heel toward your right buttock. Grasp your right foot with your right hand and pull up. Hold this stretch for a full minute. Then repeat on the other side.

  To cool down after exercising, slow down to an easy walk and gradually reduce your pace for 2–3 minutes. Then repeat the stretches just described.

- *Step 3:* Strengthen the quadricep muscles. Sit in an upright, straight-backed chair with legs uncrossed and feet flat on the floor. Raise the chair, or the chair seat, until your heels are about 1 inch clear of the floor. Begin by bending your left knee and raising your left leg about two-thirds of the way toward a horizontal position. Take 3 seconds to raise the leg, hold in the raised position for 3 seconds, then lower back to the floor for three3nds. Repeat 10 times in all. Then repeat with your right leg.

Almost everyone can do this simple unweighted exercise. But to build strength, you must raise your leg against resistance. Resistance can be an ankle weight or a plastic bag or fanny pack filled with sand, or a bag of frozen peas, or a heavy boot with a small weight attached. Place the weight on your foot, and raise your leg against the resistance of the weight. As your quadricep muscles become stronger, keep increasing the weight. Eventually, you should be able to do 3 or 4 sets of 10 repetitions each. Regardless of how strong your quadriceps become, do not raise your leg more than two-thirds of the way toward the horizontal.

However, the best way to do leg extension exercises is to use a Nautilus knee-thigh machine that offers both leg extension and leg curling equipment. Almost every gym or health spa has one of these machines.

- *Step 4:* Strengthen the hamstring muscles. Stand upright facing a door, chair, or any kind of firm support and hold on to it. Place your weight on your left leg. Then bend back your right knee so that your right heel moves toward your right buttock. Raise your right leg only to the horizontal position. Take 3 seconds to raise your foot, hold in the horizontal position for 3 seconds, then lower back to the floor for 3 seconds. Do 10 repetitions with your right foot, then 10 repetitions with your left.

It should take only a few seconds to learn the movements. Next add some resistance by using ankle weights or the various makeshift weights suggested in step 3. Again, the one best way to strengthen the quadricep muscles is to use a Nautilus-type knee-thigh machine.

By strengthening and stretching both quadricep and hamstring muscles, muscle balance is restored, and in many cases, knee pain diminishes or disappears. If your chondromalacia resulted from the impact of running or racewalking, consider switching to a nonimpact exercise such as bicycling or swimming.

■ PAIN ON THE INSIDE OF THE KNEE

Discomfort on the inside of the knee is often due to stress from the shock of jarring impact caused by overuse. Obviously, you should cut back on exercising to the point where pain is not experienced. You then need to increase the shock-absorbing power of your quadricep and hamstring muscles by strengthening them through the same exercises described in Painstopper #72.

You may also help to relieve pain on the inside of the knee by wearing well-cushioned shoes.

Incidentally, pain *behind* the knee is often due to a tight hamstring muscle. It can often be relieved by using the hamstring stretch described in Painstopper #72 (step 2).

If these exercises fail to lessen your knee pain, your problem may be due to pronation (inward rolling) or supination (outward rolling) of your foot as you walk. Over-the-counter or prescription orthotics will often help knee pain that does not respond to strength-building exercises.

FOOT AND LEG PAIN

The majority of foot pains are due to wearing tight, narrow shoes or high heels or cheap, discount store shoes. To ensure buying shoes that are sufficiently large, take a brisk 40-minute walk in the late afternoon wearing a pair of moderately thick, comfortable socks inside your walking shoes. This will swell your feet to maximum size. Only then should you head for a shoe store. Once there, choose a shoe for comfort rather than style. Buy a pair of quality athletic fitness walking shoes with shock-absorbing cushioning, a wide toe box, and a firm heel. Were all Americans to wear footwear like this, at least half of all foot aches and pains would clear up spontaneously.

■ HEEL PAIN

The most common cause of chronic heel pain is due to inflammation of the plantar fascia, a band of tissue stretched like a bowstring between the heel and the base of the toes. Stress from overuse—such as running, jumping, or excessive inward rolling of the foot when walking—causes the fascia to tear away from the heel, inflaming the entire heel area and arch of the foot.

PAINSTOPPER #73:
Natural Relief for Chronic Heel Pain

If the pain is worse when you first get out of bed and stand on your heel, it's a good indication that you have plantar fasciitis (inflammation of the plantar fascia).

Usually, the pain moderates as you walk around. But it will return again if you sit for a prolonged period. And it gradually worsens with time.

It's essential to have your foot examined by a podiatrist (foot specialist) or a physician to eliminate the possibility that your heel pain may be due to a stress fracture. Assuming it is diagnosed as plantar fasciitis, the following action-steps should help relieve the pain. And if you maintain these steps for several months, they may also help the plantar fascia to recover completely.

- *Step 1:* Apply ice to the painful heel and arch area for 20 minutes twice a day. An easy way to do this is to locate a pair of old, medium-weight socks. Put both socks on your painful foot, one on top of the other. Then insert crushed ice between the socks so that about 1 inch of ice is packed against the painful heel and arch.

   Apply ice for no more than two days after the injury occurs.

- *Step 2:* Whether you normally walk, jog, or dance for exercise, reduce by one-half your normal use of your painful foot. Get your exercise by bicycling or swimming instead. Give your foot a real rest for up to six weeks. Once your heel feels better and thoroughly rested, gradually work back into your original exercise. You'd be smart, however, to avoid any excessive impact such as jumping, rope skipping, or aerobic dancing.

- *Step 3:* Prevent a taut Achilles tendon from pulling your heelbone up and back by stretching the Achilles tendon in the calf of your painful foot. Stretch it by standing on a step with your weight on the balls of your feet and your heels protruding out over the edge of the step. Now shift your weight to your heels and allow your heels to sink. This provides a good stretch for the Achilles tendon in each leg.

  For a still-better stretch, remove your good foot from the step so that your entire weight is on the ball of your painful foot. This will stretch the Achilles tendon of your painful foot still more. Hold each stretch for a full minute. Then stand normally. If a step is not available, you can stand on a piece of 4-inch × 4-inch lumber or on a thick book. It's best to stretch after warming up with a few minutes of walking. Do the Achilles stretch at least once a day.

- *Step 4:* Wear only a good-quality pair of athletic fitness walking shoes with good shock-absorbent cushioning and arch support. A pair of quality jogging shoes would do in a pinch. But cheap shoes lack the arch support necessary to prevent the inward-rolling motion of your foot while walking. If this is not immediately possible, consider buying a pair of arch supports or shock-absorbing heel pads, or molded shoe inserts for your present shoes. Don't even *think* about wearing high heels. If you must wear business shoes, buy a pair of "street walkers"—shock-absorbing athletic shoes with a polished leather finish. No one will know that you are wearing athletic training shoes.

If these steps do not lessen your heel pain in a week or so, you should see a podiatrist.

■ VARICOSE VEINS

Varicose veins are a painful degenerative condition that arises from a combination of sedentary living and eating a high-fat, low-fiber diet.

PAINSTOPPER #74:
How to Soothe the Pain of Varicose Veins

The following action-steps can help to relieve immediate pain and to prevent further varicose veins in the future.

- *Step 1:* Immediately when you wake up, and before getting out of bed, sit up in bed and stretch forward until your arms touch your toes (or reach out as far as you can). Keep your knees straight. Hold for 20 seconds or more, then release.

  Next lie on your right side. Bend your left leg back at the knee and raise your left heel toward your left buttock. Reach down with your left hand, grasp your left ankle, and pull it gently upward. Hold for 20 seconds or more, and release. Repeat with the other side.

  Then get out of bed and flex up and down on your toes for 20 times.

- *Step 2:* Whenever you feel any pain, lie down on your back. Raise one leg at a time straight up in the air as high as you can. Hold it there while you curl and wiggle your toes. Then lower it back down and repeat with the other leg. This exercise drains the venous blood while stretching the legs. This exercise will also relieve pain if you wake up during the night. You can, of course, repeat the exercise as many times as you like.

- *Step 3:* Whenever you are sitting or lying down, raise your feet 6 inches above your body and curl your toes at frequent intervals.

- *Step 4:* To relieve pain during sleep, raise the foot of your mattress 6 inches.

- *Step 5:* Take a warm-to-hot tub bath for 15–20 minutes once a day. Fill the tub until the water is 6 inches above your hips and maintain the temperature at 100 – 104° Fahrenheit. After relaxing in the warm water for a few minutes, raise one leg as high as you can and hold it there for 15–20 seconds while you curl and uncurl your toes. Keep the leg as straight as possible. Then lower it and repeat with the other leg. Raise and lower one leg each minute while you are in the tub. A few minutes before getting out, cool the water to 100° F. As soon as you get out, dry the varicose veins by toweling toward your heart.

- *Step 6:* Avoid rubbing or massaging varicose veins and never use an electric vibrator. Avoid standing continuously in any one position. Avoid constricting blood vessels by wearing elastic garters or bands on the thighs or legs. Avoid wearing high-heeled shoes or any shoes that are not made for serious walking.

- *Step 7:* Most sports therapists recommend wrapping the foot, ankle, and lower leg in a 2- to 4-inch elastic or Ace® bandage to keep the veins compressed and to prevent them from filling with blood. While the legs are wrapped, you should walk as much as possible. This helps to develop and strengthen the muscles that contract and pump blood through the veins and back to the heart.

- *Step 8:* If you are able, begin a gradual but increasing program of daily exercise, preferably walking. For details, see Painstopper #2: Walk Away from Pain. Alternatively, you can bicycle. Leg exercise is essential, not only to help ease the immediate pain but to develop the pumping action of the veins and to prevent more vein damage in the future. A lifelong program of daily walking should prevent further varicose veins for as long as you live. If you have any difficulty walking, consider walking in a swimming pool while immersed waist deep in water. Several physical therapists have recommended walking backward in water as a therapy for varicose veins. Apparently, walking backward develops seldom-used muscles that help to constrict and pump blood through sagging veins.

- *Step 9:* You can help speed recovery from varicose veins and prevent any further recurrence, by changing to a high-fiber, low-fat diet for life. Include plenty of oranges, bananas, green leafy vegetables, and shredded carrots in your diet. For a complete guide to healthful eating, look up Painstopper #3: The One Diet that Does it All. Some nutritionists also recommend taking a daily supplement of vitamin E. Bioflavonoid supplements may also help. Both are available in health food stores.

These action-steps are intended to relieve the pain of varicose veins. None is likely to repair or reverse varicose veins. But if you make these steps a permanent part of your life-style, they may gradually help to improve mild cases of varicose veins.

■ INGROWING TOENAIL

PAINSTOPPER #75:
Ending the Pain of an Ingrowing Toenail

An ingrowing toenail invariably occurs on the big toe and is usually due to wearing tight, narrow shoes or to cutting the nail incorrectly. If the toe throbs, it is probably infected and you should see a physician or podiatrist.

Cutting a V in the nail, an old folk remedy, is not recommended nowadays. The action-steps that follow describe a better way.

- *Step 1:* Ease the pain and soften the nail by soaking the foot in a bucket or footbath of comfortably hot water containing Epsom salts.

- *Step 2:* While still soft, cut the toenail straight across. Do not follow the usual curve and do not cut the nail back behind the tip of the toe.

- *Step 3:* With the tip of a wooden toothpick, insert a small piece of sterilized cotton between the toenail and flesh on each side of the toenail. Try to get the cotton under the toenail as well as the side. Don't, of course, do anything that hurts.

- *Step 4:* If the pain continues, wear open-toe sandals or cut a hole for the toenail in an old shoe.

If, after several days, the pain persists, see a podiatrist or physician.

■ BUNIONS

PAINSTOPPER #76:
How to Tame Bunion Pain

A bunion is a painful lump near the ball of the foot caused by abnormal movement of bones behind the big toe. In some people, a bunion may be the first symptom of rheumatoid arthritis. So if yours is hot, red, or swollen, see a doctor without delay. However, if it's just a plain or garden-type bunion, these simple action-steps may tame the pain.

- *Step 1:* Ice can often numb the nerves that set off the bunion pain. Wrap an icebag in a single layer of cloth and apply to the bunion site for 20 minutes every evening.

- *Step 2:* Another way to soothe an inflamed bunion is to mix some Epsom salts into a gallon of lukewarm water. Soak the bunion in the water for 20 minutes. Do not use this step on the same day as step 1.

- *Step 3:* Get yourself a pair of wide, roomy athletic fitness walking shoes with a wide toe box. And from now on wear only shoes designed for serious walking. Never wear narrow, pointed shoes or shoes with high heels.

- *Step 4:* Even with comfortable shoes, you may want to protect the bunion with a bunion cushion while walking. Or you could use a bunion bandage that fits over, and protects, the big toe. These foot aids are available in most drugstores.

If the pain persists, consult a podiatrist.

■ ACHING FEET

PAINSTOPPER #77:
Aching Feet—And How to Relieve Them

Aching feet are generally due to a combination of hammertoes, fallen arches, and rigid, flat feet. You can relieve the discomfort by doing the following exercises designed to increase the strength and flexibility of your feet and toes. All are done barefoot. Take a short rest between each step.

- *Step 1:* Lay an open towel on the floor. Stack 5 pounds of weights or books at one end. Then sit in a chair and use your toes to grasp and pull the other end of the towel toward you.

- *Step 2:* Place the balls of both feet on a stair or step so that your heels protrude backward over the edge. Keep your feet together. Hold on to something for support. Lower your heels as far as you can, then raise as high as you can until standing on tiptoe. Repeat 10–12 times. As you gain strength, do the same exercises using only one foot.

- *Step 3:* Sit in an upright chair and raise the seat so that your heels are clear of the floor. Place an ankle weight over the lower part of your aching foot. Bending at the knee, raise the lower leg and foot about two-thirds of the way toward the horizontal. You may know this exercise as a leg extension. Use enough weight to provide some resistance to your thigh muscle and increase the weight as you gain strength. To equalize muscle development, repeat the same exercise with your other foot.

- *Step 4:* Sit in the same chair at normal seat height. Grasp a pencil on the floor with your toes and raise your foot as high as you can.

- *Step 5:* Place some marbles on the floor. Use your toes to pick them up, one at a time, until you can hold half a dozen in the toes of one foot.

NECK, SHOULDER, AND UPPER BACK PAIN

If you're one of several million Americans plagued by chronic stiffness and aching in the neck, shoulders, and upper back, take heart. In most cases, the pain is due to nothing more than muscular tension caused by stress. For a whole-person approach, I recommend using Painstoppers #2, #9, and #21 to phase out the stress, which is the underlying cause of the pain. Additionally, you should use one or more of the following physical action-steps, each of which is specifically designed for relieving chronic pain and stiffness in the neck, shoulders, or upper back.

Before using any of these painstopper techniques, you should have your neck, back, or shoulder pain diagnosed by a physician or orthopedist. That's because the pain *could* be due to a whiplash accident, osteoarthritis, cervical spondylitis, myofascial syndrome, or a spinal disc problem. Once your doctor gives you medical clearance, this indicates that your neck pain is probably due to tightening of the scalene, splenii, or trapezius muscles in the neck and shoulder area. The following painstoppers have proven highly effective at relieving this type of muscular pain.

You can help to speed your recovery by not sleeping on a thick pillow or soft mattress. Use a small, flat pillow and a firm mattress. Keep your neck warm at all times and use a muffler if necessary, even during sleep. Avoid thrusting your head and jaw out forward while doing things. And stand straight and erect when you walk. Slouching stresses the spine because it, also, thrusts the head and jaw forward. Avoid sleeping on your stomach because it forces you to twist your head to one side. Finally, if you read in bed, use cushions to keep yourself as upright as you can.

PAINSTOPPER #78:
Relieving Pain in the Middle of the Back

Pain in the middle of the back is most often due to tension and inflammation in the psoas (*so-ass*) or hip flexor muscles. It can usually be relieved by the following stretching routine. Breathe regularly throughout.

- *Step 1:* Stand upright with feet together and parallel. Slide the right foot forward about 12 inches and the left foot backward for a similar distance. Keep the toes pointed forward throughout.

- *Step 2:* Raise your right arm overhead. Keep the left arm at your side.

- *Step 3:* Bend your right (forward) knee to an angle of 45 degrees (but not more).

- *Step 4:* Lean the torso back and bend the spine moderately backward so that your head and upraised arm tilt back about 10 degrees. You can bend back more if it feels comfortable. Hold 10 seconds, then release.

Then repeat on the other side. This gives a good stretch to the psoas muscles on both sides of your back.

PAINSTOPPER #79:
Melt Away Neck Pain with Temperature Therapy

A "crick in the neck" is how many of us describe a sudden muscle tear that results in extreme stiffness in the neck, making it painful to move the head. You can usually relieve the pain, and free up your neck, by applying cold or heat in the following ways.

- *Step 1:* During the first 24 hours, apply only cold to the painful spot. Either use a cold gel pack or wrap ice in a plastic bag. Insert one layer of thin towel between the ice or pack and the flesh. Keep the coldpack in place until the pain is numbed. However, do not apply cold for longer than 20 minutes at a time. You can reapply the coldpack several times a day.

- *Step 2:* Instead of, or in addition to, step 1, massage the painful area with an ice cube held in your fingers. Use a gentle, circular motion.

- *Step 3:* After 24 hours, if the pain still persists, try applying heat with your shower head. Direct the shower nozzle at the sore area of your neck. After several minutes, begin rubbing the sore area with the fingertips of your three middle fingers as you continue to spray it with water. The water should be as hot as you can stand without discomfort. Maintain the massage for several minutes. Continue to spray the top and back of your head, neck, and shoulders with the warm water for a total of 15–20 minutes.

- *Step 4:* If neither cold nor heat relieves your painful neck completely, apply alternating hot and cold showers. Do not apply heat and cold during the first 24 hours; apply cold only. After 24 hours, you can apply heat alone, or if that doesn't help, the combination of heat and cold described next.

  Spray the painful area with hot water from a showerhead for 5 minutes followed by 5 minutes of briskly cool water. You can repeat this cycle once more for a total of 20 minutes of temperature therapy. You can give one 20-minute heat-cold treatment each hour until the pain subsides. During the hot cycle, use water that is as hot as possible without causing discomfort, and during the cold cycle, use water that is as cool as possible without causing discomfort or shocking the body.

During the warm shower cycle, you can knead and massage muscles in your neck and shoulders. You can also turn and rotate your head and neck as much as possible without causing discomfort.

Applying heat and cold alternately constricts and dilates blood vessels in the neck and shoulders. This causes them to transport more blood and oxygen to muscles in the neck, thus relieving any pain.

PAINSTOPPER #80:
Relief for Sore Neck Muscles

These techniques will stretch and release excessively tight neck muscles that may be causing soreness and pain.

- *Step 1:* Place the palm of the right hand on the right shoulder and the palm of the left hand on the left shoulder.

- *Step 2:* Raise the elbows up to the horizontal position. Then,

    Push the elbows all the way back. Hold 10 seconds, and release.

    Circle the elbows 5 times one way and 5 times the other way.

    Then drop the arms back to your sides in preparation for step 3.

- *Step 3:* Hold your right arm straight out in front at shoulder height. Grasp your right elbow with your left hand. Pull the right elbow toward the left shoulder as far as you can. Hold 10 seconds, and release. Repeat on the other side.

You can repeat all three steps several times.

PAINSTOPPER #81:
Stretch Away Neck Pain

Chronic neck pain is often caused by holding a telephone under the chin for a prolonged period, or by looking down all day at a desk. It can usually be relieved by sitting in a straight-backed chair and doing the following stretches.

- *Step 1:* Drop the head all the way forward, then raise it up and back as far as you can. Repeat 5 more times.

- *Step 2:* Place the left hand on top of the head with the fingers extending down over the right side of the head and over the right ear. Gently pull the head down toward your left shoulder as far as you can without causing discomfort. Hold 10 seconds, and release. Repeat on the right side. Then repeat twice more on each side.

- *Step 3:* Turn your head all the way to the right. Then

   Raise and tilt your head back as far as possible so that the tip of your nose points up into the air.

   Without stopping, continue to move your head down and to the left so that your head is level once more and you are looking all the way back and over your left shoulder.

   Continue moving your head to face forward, then drop it all the way down.

   Continue moving your head up and to the right until you are back in the starting position, with your head turned all the way to the right.

   You have now come full circle. Circle your head twice more in the same direction, then three more times in the opposite direction.

PAINSTOPPER #82:
How to Relieve Stiff, Aching Neck and Shoulder Muscles

The following action-steps should relieve most neck and shoulder pains caused by stress and tension.

- *Step 1:* Slowly tense all the muscles in your neck and shoulders while you also stick out your jaw and raise your shoulders as high as you can toward your ears. Hold 6 seconds, and release. Repeat 4 more times.

- *Step 2:* Hold your arms out at your sides with the right palm up and the left palm down.

Turn your head all the way to the right so that you are looking at your upturned right palm.

Flip your hands over so that your left palm is now facing up. Turn your head all the way to the left so that you are looking at your upturned left palm.

Flip the hands 9 more times and turn your head and eyes as far as you can each time.

- *Step 3:* Stand erect with arms hanging loosely as your sides. Thrust your shoulders back as far as possible. Hold 10 seconds, and release.

- *Step 4:* From the same position, thrust your shoulders as far forward as possible. Hold 10 seconds, and release.

- *Step 5:* Roll shoulders forward in a circle 5 times, then roll them backward in the opposite direction 5 times. Roll your shoulders in as wide a circle as possible.

- *Step 6:* Roll one shoulder in a forward circle while you roll the other in a backward circle. Then make 5 circles in the opposite direction. Roll your shoulders in as wide a circle as possible.

If, after using all these action-steps, your neck, shoulders, and back continue to feel stiff and ache, you should see a physician or orthopedist.

NEURAL PAIN

Neural, or nerve, pain is usually caused by a virus or infection, or by nerve damage resulting from an injury (and known as causalgia), or from a vitamin deficiency. Much nerve damage is irreparable, and the pain may be lifelong. The pain itself is often excruciating, ranging from a continual burning sensation to a periodic sharp burst that may occur from once every 30 seconds to once every 3 hours or more.

Typical neural dysfunctions such as trigeminal neuralgia, tic douleureux, herpes zoster shingles, sympathetic dystrophy, or sciatica are notoriously painful. While modern over-the-counter or prescription drugs can now soothe some of the agony of neural pain, many people are unable to use these medications due to disturbing side effects, or the drugs may not work for them.

Any type of neural pain must be checked out and diagnosed by a doctor or neurologist. However, if medical treatment cannot relieve your pain, then here are several nonmedical action-steps that, it is claimed, have helped alleviate or stop neural pain for literally hundreds of Americans. As always, I caution you to have your physician's specific approval before using any action-steps in this book for the relief of chronic pain.

PAINSTOPPER #83:
Alleviating Nerve Pain by Relieving Possible Nutritional Deficiencies

A deficiency of certain B vitamins, together with vitamins C and D, have been identified as a possible cause of several very painful nerve disorders. Obviously, if your pain is due to an infection or injury, taking vitamins may not help very much. Yet having a sufficiency of B vitamins, and vitamin C and D, in the bloodstream certainly can't hurt.

I'm not talking about taking megadoses of these vitamins but merely following the manufacturer's recommendation on the label. In moderate amounts, these vitamins are cheap, and they can benefit the body in many ways.

Several small studies have linked the deficiency of the B vitamins inositol, thiamin, and B-12 with nerve damage that, in turn, may cause severe pain. One study at the VA Medical Center in Birmingham, Alabama, was made on 20 patients suffering from neuritis (nerve inflammation) associated with long-term diabetes. This type of neuritis seldom improves naturally.

Yet within seven days of starting to eat a diet high in inositol, 19 of the 20 patients obtained significant relief from their neuritis pain. When the same 20 patients were then given a diet low in inositol, their neuritis pain returned.

Although no additional studies have been reported, some researchers tend to think that, by extension, a high-inositol diet may also relieve other types of neuritis or nerve pain. In any case, foods high in inositol tend to be very good for you.

Foods High in Inositol

Most types of peas and beans have a high inositol content. During the study, researchers used fresh, dried, and canned great northern beans, canned red kidney beans, canned rutabagas, and canned navy beans. Also high in inositol are stone-ground whole-wheat flour and bread made exclusively from this flour as are also fresh cantaloupes, oranges, and grapefruit, and fresh or frozen unsweetened orange or grapefruit juice and concentrate. These foods may also contain thiamin and vitamin C.

Since B vitamins work more effectively when taken together, many nutritionists recommend taking a vitamin B complex nutritional supplement each day that includes inositol, thiamin, and B_{12}. Among foods high in B vitamins is brewer's yeast. You can take 2–3 tablespoons of brewer's yeast with your breakfast cereal or mix 2 tablespoons in a glass of orange juice each day.

You can also increase your uptake of vitamin C by eating more fresh fruits and vegetables or by taking 500 mg of ascorbic acid daily in supplement form. Supplementary vitamin D is also available in health food stores.

By boosting your intake of these vitamins, you may possibly experience pain relief similar to that reported by the neuritis patients in the Alabama study.

PAINSTOPPER #84:
An Easy Way to Minimize Neuritis Pain

Many people have reported relieving neuritis pain like this:

Mix some Epsom salts in a hot tub. Then soak in the tub with your neuritis area submerged for a full hour. Keep the water as hot as you can while remaining comfortable.

After 60 minutes, get out and take a cool-brisk shower for 2–3 minutes. The shower should feel invigorating and briskly cold, but it should not feel freezing or cold enough to shock the body.

Give yourself a brisk rubdown with a coarse towel and rest in bed for 10–15 minutes.

Herpes Zoster Shingles

Herpes zoster shingles is a virus-caused neuritis condition that generally occurs on the back or chest. It can be very painful in older people.

Although seldom fatal, the virus damages the fast nerve fibers that carry touch sensations capable of closing the pain gate. In herpes zoster, the pain gate is left wide open to pain impulses that emanate from nerve root damage caused by the virus.

Eventually, the virus subsides but only to be replaced by an equally painful condition known as postherpetic neuralgia. Doctors treat the condition with antidepressants and tranquilizers, but as all too many people have discovered, these medications may induce a variety of adverse side effects.

PAINSTOPPER #85:
Natural Ways to Relieve the Pain of Herpes Zoster Shingles

Lydia B., a 65-year-old retired nurse, lives in rural Texas. Lydia used to suffer excruciating pain from herpes zoster blisters on her back. Because of an allergy, she was unable to use a popular pain-soothing cream that is often prescribed for herpes zoster nowadays. And she found that the side effects of prescription medications were often as bad as the herpes pain itself.

But Lydia belonged to a network of people who experimented with herbs and other natural therapies. Through their newsletter, she learned that a number of members had achieved relief from herpes zoster pain by nonmedical means. By putting together their individual findings, Lydia came up with the following natural therapies.

- *Step 1:* Mix a cup of sodium bicarbonate in a bucket of water at room temperature. Then add ice cubes until the water feels briskly cool. The water temperature does not have to be freezing, but it should feel distinctly cold.

  Wring out a thick towel, or compress, in the water and apply it to the painful area. Wring out and reapply the compress every few minutes to keep it cool. Keep the water in the bucket cool by adding a few ice cubes. Keep applying until the pain disappears, or for a maximum time of 45 minutes.

- *Step 2:* Take 500 mg of the amino acid lysine orally each day and 200 units daily of vitamin E—both are available in health food stores. You should also ensure an adequate intake of vitamins B and C (see

Painstopper #83). According to members of Lydia's network, these nutritional steps gradually reduced the pain of herpes zoster.

- *Step 3:* Slice a leaf of the aloe vera plant and rub the juice into the painful herpes zoster rash or blisters. When she used up all her fresh aloe vera leaves, Lydia used aloe vera cream, obtainable in health food stores. Some network members also rubbed on vitamin E oil, which they squeezed from nutritional capsules.

While various members of the network claimed that these remedies helped reduce their herpes zoster pain, we must remember that each remedy is anecdotal and none has been tested in careful studies. Still, since they appear to have relieved pain for Lydia and her correspondents, you may like to try them also.

■ TIC DOULEUREUX

The leading cause of pain-provoked suicide, tic douleureux is considered the most agonizing pain that a human can experience. A related condition known as trigeminal, or trifacial, neuralgia is almost as terrifying. Both the tic and neuralgia arise when pressure or cold on the face and mouth sets off trigger points connected to the trigeminal nerve in the face. Fierce paroxysms of pain shoot across the face, lasting from a few seconds to several minutes. The pain may occur several times each day or only in isolated instances.

Drugs are now available to prevent the tic and neuralgia, but each has a depressing list of adverse side effects. However, circumstances linked to the pain provide a tip-off to a possible natural prophylactic. Through discovering that these pains almost always occur in sedentary people aged over 60, and seldom in fit, healthy people of normal weight, the following painstopper technique was developed.

PAINSTOPPER #86:
A Life-style Change That May End the Pain of Tic Douleureux

Although no specific studies have been done to prove it, experience shows that most people willing to take a brisk daily walk of 3 miles or more—and to maintain it for life—often obtain complete and lasting relief from the pain of tic douleureux or trigeminal neuralgia.

Alternatively, several brisk 15-minute walks taken at intervals throughout the day have also proved effective. For more about the pain-relieving effects of walking, see Painstopper #2: Walk Away from Pain

PAINSTOPPER #87:
A Simple Do-It-Yourself Massage May Defuse the World's Fiercest Pain

Taking only a few minutes, this simple massage may help to prevent any kind of facial tic, including the dreaded tic douleureux. You can use it to massage your face several times a day as a prophylactic measure. Be careful not to press on any known trigger points that might set off tic douleureux.

- *Step 1:* Place your open palms under your chin with the fingers on the lower part of your face.

- *Step 2:* Sweep your hands firmly up to your forehead and continue on up and back over the scalp. Press just firmly enough to move the skin and underlying tissue upward.

- *Step 3:* Repeat 12 times in all, and do the exercise several times a day.

SINUSITIS PAIN

It's not often that a doctor prescribes home care to relieve pain. But that's what happened after Marcia T. consulted her physician about recurring episodes of facial pain and headache. The diagnosis was chronic sinusitis, or inflammation of the membranes lining the nasal cavities above the eyes and behind the cheeks.

The pain was particularly severe when she first woke up in the morning, or whenever she bent her head forward and down. It was a pounding pain on the left side of her face that reached all the way from her teeth and nose up to her eyes and forehead and back to her ear. Marcia's nose was so completely blocked that she could breathe only through her mouth. Her speech sounded nasal, and she felt as though her head might explode at any minute.

Although sinusitis is frequently caused by a bacterial infection following a head cold, antibiotics prescribed by her doctor didn't seem to help. Nor did antihistamines, powerful decongestants, or even steroids. While he was investigating other possible causes, the physician described four non-medical ways by which Marcia could soothe her exhausting sinusitis pain.

But first, the doctor cautioned Marcia not to ignore any need for medical treatment.

"Anyone with what appears to be a cold in the head that worsens after a week should see a doctor," he explained. "Bacteria or virus from a cold or infection can creep into the sinus spaces, causing inflammation of the membranes that line these cavities. This blocks the normal mucus drainage. It traps the bacteria-laden mucus in the sinuses and creates painful pressure around the eyes, cheeks, and forehead. Anyone with a heavy mucus discharge from the nose, and down the back of the throat, that turns green or yellow, and has a thick consistency, may well have sinusitis."

The doctor explained that sinusitis may also be triggered by allergies, air pollution, airborne irritants, smoking, a food sensitivity—especially to milk—or a structural abnormality such as a deviated septum. If not medically checked out, chronic sinusitis could lead to asthma.

Meanwhile, here is how her doctor recommended that Marcia relieve her sinus headache pain.

PAINSTOPPER #88:
Chase Away Sinusitis Pain Naturally

- *Step 1:* Inhale steam. To soothe sinus pain quickly, cover the head with a towel and inhale steam from a basin of hot water. Some people prefer to inhale the steam from the spout of a kettle of boiling water. Naturally, you must be very, *very* careful because steam is *hot* and you can burn yourself. Some people add salt to the hot water. As a second-choice alternative, you can sit in a shower or bathroom and allow a spray of steaming hot water to run from the shower head. Again, be very careful not to contact the hot water but to merely inhale the steam and moist heat. However, the water has to be really hot for this to work.

- *Step 2:* Apply moist heat directly. After inhaling moist heat, as in step 1, apply 20 minutes of moist heat directly to the top of your face and forehead, wherever the sinus pain hurts. Use a hot pack to apply the heat. To make a hot pack, wrap a loaf of bread in a towel, immerse in hot water not exceeding 112° Fahrenheit, and wring out. Lacking a loaf of bread, use a thick towel. Then cover with a single layer of dry thin towel and apply to the painful sinus area behind the forehead, nose, and cheekbones. Again, take care not to burn yourself. Reapply the hot pack every few minutes to maintain the temperature. Almost always, this direct application of moist heat significantly cuts the pain level or may cause it to disappear altogether.

- *Step 3:* Use gentle massage. If pain still persists, use your fingertips to gently massage the painful sinus area. Massage the cheeks and forehead above and below the eyes and rub the cheeks over your teeth. Use a circular motion and apply a firm but gentle pressure. Rub only on the flat parts of your face that are underlain by bone and stay far away from the eye sockets and eyes.

- *Step 4:* Avoid irritating the sinuses. To reduce pain of sinusitis, stay indoors in a room with an even temperature and add moisture with a vaporizer or humidifier. Keep the relative humidity between 45 and 65 percent. Avoid smoking and alcohol, or exposure to dust, pollen, or very dry air. And avoid blowing your nose hard. It could force more bacteria into the sinuses. Finally, drink plenty of fluids to help prevent mucus from congesting and blocking the nasal passages.

Using these four steps enabled Marcia to bring her pain under control swiftly and to reduce it to manageable levels. Eventually, her doctor found that an allergy to cows' milk was causing Marcia's painful condition.

HEMORRHOID PAIN

Hemorrhoids are varicose veins of the anal canal, and fully 50 percent of Americans aged over 40 have some degree of hemorrhoidal discomfort or irritation. The cause is eating the standard American diet, that is, a low-fiber diet high in fat, flesh foods, dairy products, and refined carbohydrates (primarily white flour, white bread, and sugar). Such a low-residue diet produces small, hard feces that cause straining during a bowel movement. When this exertion is coupled with holding the breath, hemorrhoidal veins form in the anus area. Straining at stool is made worse by a sedentary life-style, chronic coughing due to smoking, consuming alcohol, being overweight, and lifting heavy weights improperly.

The causes of hemorrhoids were identified by comparing Americans with blacks living in rural areas of Africa. In rural Africa, where hemorrhoids are virtually unknown, the population lives almost entirely on a high-fiber diet of whole grains, fresh fruits and vegetables, legumes, nuts, and seeds. Native black Africans also tend to be lean, fit, and much more active physically than the average American.

The swelling of hemorrhoids causes discomfort and irritation that ranges from pain during bowel movements to a severe itching after wiping the anal area with toilet paper. Attacks commonly last for several days and then subside. A badly inflamed hemorrhoid may bulge out through the anus and have to be pushed back after each bowel movement.

Usually, the first indication is a bright red blood spot on toilet paper. (By contrast, blood from the stomach or small intestine causes a black, tarry stool.)

However, *any* type of rectal bleeding requires medical diagnosis. Severe hemorrhoids can lead to a painful anal fissure for which surgery is the only answer. Nowadays, even the most severe hemorrhoids can be medically removed by a choice of safe methods. These range from painless infrared coagulation—an outpatient procedure requiring no anesthesia—to rubber band ligation, injection, electric current treatment, or traditional surgery. Surgery is usually needed only when hemorrhoids protrude outside the anus.

Often enough, immediate medical treatment is not necessary. And for these cases, relief from pain and other symptoms can usually be achieved by practicing the following painstopper action-steps.

PAINSTOPPER #89:
Swift Relief from Hemorrhoidal Inflammation

Much hemorrhoidal swelling and discomfort are due to the constant downward pull of gravity. This swelling can be swiftly relieved by a simple stretch known as the knee-chest position.

- *Step 1:* Kneel on a mat or rug on the floor.

- *Step 2:* Bend forward and down so that your right shoulder, and the right side of your face, are resting on the floor. Your buttocks should now be raised in the air.

- *Step 3:* Breathe slowly and deeply as you remain in this position for as long as it feels comfortable, that is, for a maximum of several minutes.

Then repeat on your other side, with your left shoulder and the left side of your face on the floor.

PAINSTOPPER #90:
Let Moist Heat Alleviate Hemorrhoidal Discomfort

If you have a tub bath, you can reduce hemorrhoidal pain by filling the bath with 6 inches of hot water and then sitting in it for 15 minutes. The water should be as warm as possible without being uncomfortably hot. Run in more hot water if needed to maintain the temperature.

A shallow hot tub bath works by reducing the size of swollen hemorrhoidal veins while also easing any spasm of the anal sphincter muscles. Avoid adding anything to the bath water, such as salts, since it could irritate the hemorrhoids.

To shrink hemorrhoids even more effectively, try sitting in alternate hot and cold baths. For this, you'll need a sitz bath or some kind of second bath in addition to your regular tub.

Fill your tub bath with hot water as previously described. Then fill your second bath to the same height with water that feels briskly cold but that is not cold enough to cause discomfort or to shock the body.

Sit in the hot tub for 5 minutes. Then shift to the cold bath and sit in it for 1 minute. Repeat the same cycle twice more. Then towel dry.

If baths are not practical, consider applying towels, soaked in hot water and wrung out, to the anal area.

Although it does not supply moist heat, many people with hemorrhoids have found relief by sitting on a heating pad with the switch set on "low."

PAINSTOPPER #91:
A Natural Movement That Often Relieves Hemorrhoid Pain

It's never been tested in any study, but at least a dozen people have told me that they were able to relieve hemorrhoid irritation and discomfort by walking on their hands and feet.

"That means walking on all fours," one man said, "not walking on your hands and knees."

The same man advised practicing indoors on the living room floor: "Perhaps it's because our ancestors walked on all fours," he said, "but there's something about this natural movement that seems to make hemorrhoids shrink and feel a whole lot better. Walk on all fours for as long as you can, say, 10 minutes at a time. And do it several times each day. For as long as you keep this up, there's a good chance you will never be bothered by hemorrhoids again."

When I asked a physical therapist about this, he explained that all types of rhythmic or stretching exercise benefits hemorrhoids, but that weight training or weight-lifting should be avoided. He advised that if you *must* lift a heavy weight, keep the back straight, lift by stooping, and exhale as you lift. Exerting any body muscle while holding your breath can cause hemorrhoids to swell. Consuming alcohol and being overweight may also increase your risk of getting hemorrhoids.

PAINSTOPPER #92:
Long-Term Relief for Hemorrhoid Problems

A high-fiber diet is an essential step in achieving permanent freedom from hemorrhoid pain. Even if you have your present hemorrhoids surgically removed, they may reappear if you continue to eat a low-fiber diet, to avoid exercise, and to be overweight.

To get started, follow the advice in Painstopper #3: The One Diet That Does It All. This action-step describes how to replace all or most of the flesh foods, eggs, dairy products, refined carbohydrates, and other unhealthy, low-fiber foods in your diet with plant-based foods bursting with fiber. By making this one dietary switch, your stools will change from small, hard feces to larger, softer feces that pass much more easily through the anal passage. This same diet will also help you lose weight, another desirable step in remaining hemorrhoid-free.

Admittedly, it may take you a week or two to phase in a high-fiber diet. In the meantime, you can soften your stools by adding 3 tablespoons of unprocessed bran to your breakfast cereal and 3 more to your dinner. Bran is such an effective stool-softener that a study in Denmark (reported in the *British Medical Journal,* May 3, 1986) found that, when combined with several daily sitz baths, it relieved anal fissure pain better than prescription medicated ointment. And anal fissure pain is usually worse than hemorrhoidal pain. In the study, each participant took a 15-minute sitz bath each morning and evening and after each bowel movement.

Until you have fully adopted the diet in Painstopper #3, another way to avoid straining at stool is to lubricate the anal canal with either plain petroleum jelly (Vaseline) or an OTC hemorrhoid cream. Use your fingers to spread the lubricant inside the anus and wash your hands carefully afterward. This helps ease hard, low-fiber stools through the anal canal. However, once you have fully adopted the diet in Painstopper #3, your stools should become permanently soft and easily passed.

You can also help to keep stools soft by drinking eight 8-ounce glasses of water, or other nonalcoholic fluid, daily.

SCIATICA PAIN

"It's a sharp, shooting, cutting pain that radiates all the way from my buttocks down the back of my right thigh and leg and into my foot, and it feels as if my legbones are being crushed."

This was Jill N., a 54-year old Chicago schoolteacher, describing the pain in her leg to her orthopedist.

"The pain is often worse after sitting down, or when I make any sudden movement," she said. "Whenever I turn or bend at the waist, or bend my knee or ankle, or when I cough or sneeze or lift anything or strain at stool, there's this sudden, sharp, and severe pain the length of my leg. It's always worse at night. The only real relief I get is when I stand erect or lie down in bed."

It took the orthopedist only 3 minutes to diagnose Jill's pain as sciatica, or inflammation of the sciatic nerve. After they traverse the entire length of the spinal column, the body's five spinal nerves unite in the buttocks to become the two sciatic nerves. One sciatic nerve then radiates down the back of each thigh and leg into each foot.

Understandably, anything that impinges on the spinal nerves as they traverse the spinal column can cause severe sciatica pain in one or both legs.

As the orthopedist explained to Jill, the primary cause of sciatica is a herniated or bulging spinal disc. Other possible causes range from a tight piriformis muscle to spinal arthritis, a tumor, a back injury, scarring from back surgery, or an infection. Any of these can place pressure on the spinal nerves, which manifests as an excruciating pain in the back of the thighs and legs.

The orthopedist prescribed one day of bed rest followed by anti-inflammatory medication and aspirin. Surgery would be considered only as a last desperate resort.

But the rest and medication didn't seem to help. Gradually, Jill's right leg became so irritated and sore that it failed to stretch while walking. She found herself walking on her toes with her knees slightly bent, a position that relaxed the sciatic nerve and allowed her to walk with less pain.

A friend, who noticed Jill's painful gait, recommended a yoga instructor who specialized in relieving back pain.

"If it's not too severe, or caused by a ruptured disc or tumor, most cases of sciatica respond well to gentle yoga stretching postures," the yoga instructor told Jill. "I also recommend contrasting heat and cold therapy. And since it's often painful for people with sciatica to strain at stool, they frequently become constipated. Again, yoga has a simple answer. It's called the yoga diet."

The yoga instructor's reputation as a pain healer was well founded. Six weeks after he taught Jill some basic yoga stretches, her sciatica had almost completely vanished. Instead of hobbling along on her toes she could walk for miles with a brisk, athletic stride. And all traces of constipation were gone.

The following painstopper action-steps explain the key yoga postures and other natural therapies that helped Jill to recover completely from sciatica.

PAINSTOPPER #93:
Gentle Stretches to Soothe and End Sciatica Pain

Since all yoga stretches are a form of traction, you should avoid practicing yoga during the second half of pregnancy. And, of course, no one should use the following action-steps without first having their pain medically diagnosed.

Before beginning any stretches, take a short 5-minute walk while you swing your arms. This will warm up your muscles and make you more flexible. Then practice the following stretching postures, one by one.

STRETCH 1: The Knee-to-Chest Curl

- *Step 1:* Lie on your back on a rug on the floor with knees raised and feet about 12 inches apart.

- *Step 2:* Raise one knee and pull it into your chest with clasped hands. Bounce this knee into your chest 20 – 40 times. Then release and repeat with the other knee.

- *Step 3:* Raise both knees together and pull into your chest with clasped hands. Bounce your knees into your chest 20 – 40 times. Relax and lower your legs to the floor. Repeat 2 more times.

- *Step 4:* Raise both knees together and pull into your chest with clasped hands. Pull in your knees as close to your chest as you can. Hold this position. As you exhale, raise head, neck, and shoulders off the floor and crunch them upward. Hold 6–8 seconds or until you begin to inhale. Repeat this step a total of 5 times.

- *Step 5:* Return to your original position, lying on your back with knees drawn up and feet flat on the floor. Assuming that your right leg is painful, place your right palm on the inside of your right thigh.

  Grasp the right thigh with your palm and fingers and begin to massage and roll the flesh upward and outward, forcing the flesh up and around the thigh bone. Use light but firm pressure and avoid trying to force anything. With a little persistence, this action-step should roll the sciatic nerve back into the natural position it occupied before becoming inflamed.

STRETCH 2: The Spinal Twist

- *Step 1:* Lie on your back on a rug on the floor. Your knees should be bent and your feet flat on the floor. Keep your knees together throughout this exercise.

- *Step 2:* Keeping your arms on the floor, extend them sideways, palms down. Keep your arms, shoulders, head, and upper body flat on the floor throughout this exercise.

- *Step 3:* Keeping your knees together, bend them to the left and lower them all the way to the floor. Hold 20 seconds as you increase this stretch. Then release and return your knees to the upright position.

    Repeat on the right side by lowering your knees all the way to the floor. Hold 20 seconds while you increase the stretch. Then release and return your knees to the upright position.

Repeat twice more on each side.

STRETCH 3: The Forward Bend

This beneficial yoga posture stretches the entire spine and legs and the spinal and sciatic nerves. Often, it removes the spinal nerves from contact with any discs or bones that may be exerting pressure and causing irritation that manifests as pain in the sciatic nerves.

- *Step 1:* Remove your shoes. Sit on a rug on the floor with your legs stretched straight out on the floor in front of you.

- *Step 2:* Keeping your legs straight, reach forward with your arms and grasp your right big toe with your right hand, and your left big toe with your left hand. If you cannot reach your toes, grasp your ankles instead. Keep reaching out toward your toes and don't bend your knees. Hold this position for 60 seconds, or up to 3 minutes if you can. Continue to breathe naturally throughout.

    Then release and straighten up.

- *Step 3:* Keep your left leg straight out on the floor in front of you. Bend the knee of your right leg and draw your right heel toward you and back as far as you can into your crotch. Next drop your right knee down toward the floor. This brings the sole of your right foot against your left thigh. Keep your right heel as close to your crotch as you can. And lower your right knee as far as you can toward the floor.

    Now reach forward and grab the toes of your left foot with both hands. Continue to keep your left leg straight. If you cannot reach your left toes, grasp your left ankle instead. Keep reaching out toward your left toes as you continue to hold this position for 60 seconds, or up to 3 minutes if you can.

    Then release and return to the upright seated position.

Repeat on the other side, keeping your leg straight and bending your left knee.

PAINSTOPPER #94:
Let Thermal Therapy Ease Sciatica Pain

Since sciatica can inhibit sensitivity to heat or cold, older persons should use discretion in applying the action-steps that follow.

- *Step 1:* Sit in a sitz or hip bath, or an ordinary tub bath, filled to a depth of 10 inches with water at a temperature of 110 – 115° Fahrenheit. Put another way, the water should be as warm as possible without causing discomfort. When you are immersed, the water should not come above your waist. Add additional hot water, if necessary, to maintain the temperature while you are bathing. Relax in the bath for 10 minutes; then get out and towel yourself dry.

- *Step 2:* Contrasting hot and cold baths can provide even better results. They will often prevent or inhibit further sciatica attacks.

    To use this method, relax in a warm tub bath exactly as described in step 1. After 10 minutes, get out and take a brief cold shower. The water should feel briskly cold but should not be cold enough to cause actual discomfort or to shock the body.

Spray your entire body with the cold shower for a period of 10 – 15 seconds. Then get out. Give your body an invigorating rub-down with a rough towel as you dry off. Immediately afterward, lie down in bed, or in a warm place, and relax for 10 – 15 minutes.

Another way to provide alternate hot and cold therapy is to stand first under a warm shower. The water should be as warm as possible without causing discomfort. Play the spray on your painful buttocks, thigh, and calf areas and on your spine and lower back. Remain in the shower for up to 10 minutes.

Next switch to a cold shower as just described. Spray your entire body with the cold shower for 10 – 15 seconds. Then get out, towel yourself dry as just described, and relax in a warm place for 10 – 15 minutes.

PAINSTOPPER #95:
How a Yoga Instructor KOs Sciatica Pain

Jill's yoga instructor had some further suggestions for alleviating sciatica pain. "Ice packs," he said, "can provide powerful pain relief when applied along the course of the sciatic nerve, that is, along the back of the thigh and calf. Frozen gel packs work just as well. Place a single layer of thin, dry towel between the cold pack and the skin and hold the pack in place with an elastic bandage. Remove when the pain disappears, or after a maximum of 20 minutes."

For acute sciatica pain, the yoga instructor suggested using contrasting hot and cold packs, keeping each in place for a maximum of 20 minutes before removing. You can make a hot pack by wrapping a loaf of bread in a towel, soaking it in hot water, and wringing it out. Rewarm it several times, if necessary, to maintain the temperature. Always place a single layer of thin, dry towel between any thermal pack and your skin. You can repeat the hot-cold cycle 2 or 3 times if necessary.

Straining at stool often triggers sciatica pain. You can avoid any further need to strain by changing to the high-fiber, plant-based diet described in Painstopper #3: The One Diet That Does It All. This diet—also known as the yoga diet—results in large, soft stools that pass easily through the anal canal without requiring any straining or effort at all. For hundreds of former sciatica sufferers who have adopted this diet, constipation has become just a memory.

For painless sleep, lie on your back and place a pillow under the knee of your painful leg. During an acute sciatica attack, pack pillows all around your painful leg to prevent any movement. You may also find that bedclothes abrade and irritate the sciatic nerve. To prevent this, wear long johns or athletic tights while sleeping. By keeping your legs extra warm, they also soothe the sciatic nerve.

Chapter 13

HOW TO TAKE THE HURT OUT OF EMOTIONAL PAIN

If you've read this book up to and including Chapter 8, you'll have learned that the underlying cause of most pain is unresolved emotional stress that causes pain to originate in the body and to be experienced in the mind. So the type of pain we've been talking about so far is really body-mind pain—or what most of us know as physical pain.

So what is emotional pain? Is it real? How does it differ from body-mind pain? And can we relieve it naturally?

All the answers are "Yes." Emotional pain *is* real, it's extremely common, and it is quite different from body-mind pain.

"I'm hurting," is how Janet L. described her feelings when her handsomely embroidered quilt won only fourth prize at a local quilt show. "It's terribly unfair. My quilt was easily the best. I feel angry, resentful, and bitter about the whole thing."

This is a classical example of what we mean by emotional pain. But in reality, emotional pain is layperson's language for the mental anguish, hurt, and unhappiness that, to some degree, accompanies every negative emotion. Whether we feel lonely, bored, neglected, or frustrated — or any one of a dozen similar negative mind-states — they all cause us to feel hurt, sad, and unhappy.

We call it "emotional pain." But health professionals define it as depression or, in some cases, anxiety. So while we shall continue to use the term "emotional pain," what we're really talking about is a mild level of depression or anxiety. And yes, provided depression or anxiety are psychologically induced, it's relatively easy to relieve the hurt and sadness they invoke and to end the depression for good.

■ MOST PAINSTOPPING TECHNIQUES DON'T WORK ON EMOTIONAL PAIN

Back in Chapter 1, you were cautioned against "page shopping" or turning to a chapter halfway through this book without having read and absorbed the preceding chapters first. So unless you have already read and absorbed this book up to and including Chapter 8, you may not understand much of what I'm saying here. In this case, I suggest turning back and reading and absorbing these earlier chapters first.

Here are some key facts you need to know. First, body-mind pain occurs when physiological pressure on nerve endings in the body send pain impulses over slow nerve fibers through the neurological pain gate and on to the brain's reticular and straight-line systems where they are interpreted as physical pain.

But only body-mind pain travels by this route. When we feel anxious or depressed, the resulting emotional pain does *not* follow this pathway. For the first time in this book, we're looking at a different kind of pain, a pain or hurt that originates and is experienced entirely within the mind.

This means that most of the painstopper action-steps described in this book are ineffective against depression and anxiety.

Emotional Pain Rarely Exists Without Physical Tension and Discomfort

Second, emotional pain rarely exists by itself. Some degree of body-mind pain almost always occurs simultaneously. That's because emotional pain is merely a by-product of experiencing a negative emotion in the mind. And if you've read this book so far, you will already know what happens whenever the mind experiences any negative emotion.

When Janet L. felt angry, resentful, and bitter, her mind perceived these negative emotions as threats. So Janet's mind triggered the fight-or-flight response, a primitive reaction that placed her entire body-mind in a crisis state. One fight-or-flight mechanism kept her muscles charged with energy so that they remained tense. It wasn't long before Janet began to feel physically tense and uncomfortable.

Thus Janet was hurting not only in her mind but in her body as well.

Emotional Pain is Intensified by Distorted Thinking

What actually happened was this. Janet's mind was being programmed by fear that she might not win first prize at the quilt show—a negative belief. The effect of this fear-based belief was to distort her thinking. She thought that she had been unfairly treated. This negative thought then released the negative feelings of anger, resentment, and bitterness. The negative emotions then triggered the fight-or-flight response that caused Janet to feel physically tense and uncomfortable while she also felt mentally hurt and unhappy.

Modern psychology holds that the entire process just described explains the cause of both emotional stress and emotional pain. But emotional pain is intensified by the distorted and illogical way in which our thinking process functions whenever the mind is programmed by a negative belief.

Although most painstopper action-steps in this book *are* ineffective against emotional pain, several are *very* effective.

■ AN ANTIDOTE TO EMOTIONAL PAIN

One highly effective antidote to depression or anxiety is Painstopper #2: Walk Away from Pain. By walking briskly for 35 minutes or more, and raising your pulse and breathing rates, endorphins are released that block pain receptors in the brain. Any type of brisk, rhythmic exercise, maintained for 35 minutes or more, should also block out both body-mind *and* emotional pain—and prevent it from returning for the rest of the day. Several large studies have demonstrated that brisk aerobic exercise performed daily is one of the most effective ways to overcome depression or anxiety.

Since emotional pain is a by-product of emotional stress, it follows that any painstopper technique that defuses stress and tension will also help to defuse emotional pain.

As you will recall from reading Chapters 5 through 8, stress and tension can be relieved by a variety of therapies ranging from relaxation and biofeedback to belief restructuring. Whatever we do to alleviate stress also helps to take the hurt out of emotional pain.

I particularly recommend using

Painstopper #7: Learning to Beat Pain with Abdominal Breathing

Painstopper #8: Learning to Identify Muscular Tension

Painstopper #9: Relaxation Training—Nature's Prescription for Pain Relief

Painstopper #10: Experiencing Speedy Relief from Stress and Tension

Painstopper #11: Biofeedback Training—Mind over Pain

■ KEY ACTION-STEPS FOR HALTING EMOTIONAL PAIN

When we get down to basics, the root causes of emotional pain are

1. Programming the mind with inappropriate negative beliefs.
2. These negative beliefs then distort our thinking process, causing us to think in an illogical and unbalanced way.

Painstopper #21: Keep Pain at Bay with Positive Beliefs was specifically designed to keep our minds from being run by negative beliefs.

Likewise, Painstoppers #96, #97, and #98 describe how to overcome distorted and illogical ways of thinking that are the root cause of emotional pain.

For best results, Painstoppers #21 and #96–98 should be used in overcoming emotional pain. Since the use of Painstopper #21 has been explained in full in Chapter 8, I shall not repeat it here. I must emphasize, however, that use of this painstopper is virtually essential if you are really serious about ending your emotional pain.

■ AN EXCITING NEW TECHNIQUE FOR RELIEVING EMOTIONAL PAIN

While behavioral medicine has been revolutionizing the health care field, a similar revolution has been going on in the field of mental health. Out of the human potential movement of the past three decades have emerged a variety of New Age helping techniques for overcoming depression and anxiety.

Of these, *cognitive therapy* has proved so effective in overcoming psychologically induced depression and anxiety that it has been widely adopted by thousands of mental health professionals. At the same time, it is so simple that almost anyone can practice it at home.

If you have read the preceding chapters of this book, you will already know that the mind is really a biological computer. The software that programs our biocomputer is the values and beliefs that we hold in our minds.

Pioneering researchers like Aaron T. Beck recognized that a mind programmed with negative beliefs not only sees threats and hostility where none actually exist, but it also distorts our rational thinking process.

But it was another pioneer researcher, David D. Burns, who, while working along these lines at the University of Pennsylvania some years ago, discovered that most cases of depression were caused not by some complex biological process deep within the body, but by ten common types of distorted and illogical thinking. The psychotherapy that Dr. Burns developed out of this discovery is known today as cognitive therapy.

■ HOW DISTORTED THINKING CREATES EMOTIONAL PAIN

Using our minds irrationally is something many of us do every day. And every time we distort our thinking process, we experience some degree of depression or anxiety.

Here are ten variations of distorted thinking.

1. Making a mountain out of a molehill.
2. Exaggerating a minor drawback while ignoring an overwhelming number of advantages.
3. All or nothing thinking—seeing yourself as a total failure if your performance does not measure up in just one area, even though you may have succeeded at everything else.
4. Allowing yourself to be run by the way you feel instead of by logical thinking.

5. Prefacing statements with "I must," "I should," "I ought," or "I should not." This is an almost guaranteed way to distort your thinking process.

6. Jumping to a negative conclusion although there are no facts to support it.

7. Ignoring positive factors while you concentrate on negative points.

8. Viewing a single negative aspect as an endlessly repeated pattern of defeat.

9. Seeing yourself as responsible for something when you are not.

10. Seeing yourself and others negatively. For instance, you may label yourself as a "loser," or if someone's behavior rubs you the wrong way, you might label him as "dysfunctional"—all without any real justification.

Any one or a combination of these irrational ways of thinking can lead a person into depression, anxiety, or an associated form of emotional pain.

■ COGNITIVE THERAPY—A POWERFUL TOOL FOR HEALING EMOTIONAL PAIN

Cognitive Therapy works by teaching a depressed person to identify these distorted ways of thinking and to think in a more rational way. When this is done, most cases of psychologically induced depression and emotional pain swiftly disappear.

Cognitive therapy begins by having you look inward for the source of your emotional pain rather than outward. What you feel hurt or angry about is unimportant. It's how your mind is *processing* the information that counts.

For example, David W. bought a used car that seemed plagued with problems. First, the windshield wipers quit in the middle of a heavy rainstorm on a busy freeway. Then the car refused to start. Finally, the radio and tape player went dead. Other than this, the car seemed in unusually good condition with low mileage and plenty of pickup and power.

But David saw it otherwise.

"I've had three different breakdowns in as many days," he said angrily. "This car's just no good. I've wasted my money. It's a real lemon."

How Distorted Thinking Caused David W.'s Emotional Pain

Yet when a mechanic checked the car, he found only one thing wrong, a faulty ignition switch. This one switch had been responsible for all three failures David had experienced.

Although David had the switch replaced, he continued to believe that the car was worthless. He felt so depressed and unhappy that he consulted a psychotherapist. Right off, the therapist told David to stop thinking about the car.

"It's not the car that's making you feel hurt and depressed," the therapist said. "It's the way your mind is thinking about it."

The therapist explained that David was committing not one but several of the ten varieties of distorted thinking. For instance, he was making a mountain out of a molehill: exaggerating a minor drawback while ignoring an overwhelming number of advantages; allowing himself to be run by the way he felt, jumping to a conclusion without supporting facts, and ignoring positive points while concentrating on negative factors.

"Your mind is negatively programmed so you see the world in a distorted way," the therapist said. "Instead of seeing a safe, nonthreatening world out there, you see everything as negative and threatening."

"Your thinking is so distorted that you have blown up a single small drawback in your car into a huge generalization that the entire car is worthless," he went on. "Today it's your car. Tomorrow, it could be your job, your finances, or your relationships. Yet you don't *have* to go on feeling hurt or depressed. Through cognitive therapy you can feel any way you want to feel at any time."

Once David learned to recognize when his thinking was distorted, it took only a few weeks for all traces of his depression and emotional hurt to disappear for good.

■ ELIMINATE ILLOGICAL THINKING WITH COGNITIVE THERAPY

Painstoppers #96, #97, and #98 describe how to use the same cognitive therapy techniques that the psychotherapist taught David.

But, first, a word of caution. These techniques are safe to use provided your doctor has given you medical clearance and is satisfied that you do not have clinical or chronic low-grade depression or severe anxiety or any other physical or psychological problem, such as schizophrenia or hallucinating, that might be adversely affected by using cognitive therapy, belief restructuring, or any similar form of do-it-yourself psychotherapy. Otherwise, you should use these action-steps only with the knowledge and consent of your physician.

Again, these techniques are not intended to lessen the effects of genuine grief resulting from loss of a loved one, or any other kind of loss, for which grief provides a natural catharsis and relief. Genuine grief is not a negative emotion, and it is not regarded as emotional pain.

PAINSTOPPER #96:
Halting Emotional Pain with Stop-Go Switching

This powerful mind technique uses the same principle as the stop-go switching described in Painstopper #6. Before you can use it, however, you must prepare a positive "seed thought." The seed thought can be a mental picture of a beautiful garden, or beach or nature scene, or anything that will turn on feelings of happiness, pleasure, or pleasant memories. Scenes of lovemaking are fine. Spend a few moments choosing and putting together a scene like this. And be able to bring it into your mind instantly.

You also need to wear a loosely fitting rubber band around your left wrist (or your right wrist if you're left-handed). Or if this is not possible, pinch your wrist instead.

When you detect the first hint of emotional hurt or pain, immediately call out "Stop!" and snap your rubber band. If others are within hearing say "Stop!" silently—but give your rubber band a good vigorous snap—or pinch your wrist. Call out "Stop!" three times in all—and each time audibly snap your rubber band.

This distraction will bring your mind to a complete halt.

Stop what you're doing and, either sitting or standing, take five deep, slow belly breaths (abdominal breathing is described in Painstopper #7).

As you begin your first inhalation, call out "Go!" and snap your rubber band loudly again. Immediately upon exhaling, slide your seed thought into your mind and hold it there. If another thought intrudes, slide it off your mind and replace the seed thought.

Each time you inhale, call out "Go!" and snap your rubber band. And each time you exhale, check to see that your seed thought is still firmly in your mind. As you continue to hold the seed thought-image on your inner video screen, your emotional pain will gradually give way to the pleasant feelings associated with your seed thought.

This is not the same thing as repressing or denying a negative emotion. You fully acknowledge that a negative thought was releasing a negative emotion that was causing your emotional pain. And you recognize that it's perfectly all right to have a negative emotion. But you also realize that it's downright foolish to continue to suffer and hurt mentally when you have the power to act and replace your emotional pain with emotional pleasure.

Never forget that your mind is simply a biocomputer. Your subconscious mind will do whatever it's told to do. When you program it with a pain-provoking negative belief, such as "I never forgive a slight," your thinking is distorted, and your biocomputer kicks out a pain-causing emotion. Feed in a positive belief instead, such as "I forgive all slights," and immediately your biocomputer kicks out a positive thought that releases a positive emotion that begins to make you feel good.

When we feed garbage into our minds, we get garbage out. The stop technique effectively stops your mind from continuing to think in a distorted pattern and prepares the way for you to identify exactly what your mind was doing.

If you're at work, and don't have time to identify your distorted thinking process right now, you can end this action-step here. Otherwise, flow on without pause into Painstopper #97.

PAINSTOPPER #97:
Identify Your Distorted Thinking Patterns

The way we feel depends on the way we were recently thinking, that is, on whether our thoughts were logical or distorted.

As soon as you have calmed the mind by using Painstopper #96, recall what you were thinking about immediately before you detected the existence of emotional pain. Then analyze what your mind was *doing* with this information.

Was it thinking calmly and logically? Or was it committing one or more of the ten variations of distorted thinking (listed earlier in this chapter under "How Distorted Thinking Creates Emotional Pain")?

Suppose you recently entrusted a confidence to a close friend only to find she had repeated it to several other people. A natural reaction might be for you to say, "Betty betrayed the trust I placed in her. I'll never trust *anyone* again."

It might seem natural to feel angry, hurt, and betrayed. But to lose your faith in *everyone* is all-or-nothing thinking. You are magnifying your loss of trust in one person and generalizing it to include everyone. Also, you are allowing yourself to be run by the way you feel.

Or you might find yourself in the role of being a parent of a child who loses interest in school and begins to get poor grades. You experience emotional pain because you feel you have failed in your parental responsibilities. Actually, the child could be going through a temporary period of teenage rebelliousness. So here again, your emotional pain is due to distorted thinking, to seeing yourself as being responsible for your child's grades when you are obviously not.

Few salespeople haven't been depressed and discouraged at some point in their career. "I've made 14 calls this week without making a single sale," a young salesman told me. "This is my third week on the job. I guess I'm a born loser."

It took further questioning to learn that a typical salesperson in his field made over 600 calls each year and that just two sales a year meant affluence.

Thus most of this salesman's emotional pain was due to distorted thinking, to seeing himself negatively, and to labeling himself as a "born loser"—all without any real justification.

The mere act of identifying your pattern of distorted thinking is frequently all it takes to chase away your emotional pain. But if you'd like to go further, to learn how you can virtually eliminate emotional pain entirely, merely continue on directly into Painstopper #98.

PAINSTOPPER #98:
How to Feel Terrific Nearly All of the Time

We experience emotional pain because our culture has conditioned us to. Our culture has taught us to believe that we are not responsible for, or in control of, our thoughts and feelings.

When our culture conditions us to believe that something a person says is insulting, we will feel angry and hurt. When our culture conditions us to believe that something is unjust, we will feel resentful and hurt.

We feel angry, resentful, and hurt because our belief system tells us that we should feel this way. In other words, our culture has taught us that it's perfectly "natural" to feel hurt and upset.

Obviously, there *are* times when we should respond to an event assertively and even aggressively. But 90 percent of the time, when we respond with a negative emotion, we end up harming ourselves more than we harm anyone else. In most cases, when we're mad at someone, the other person doesn't even know. But our negative reaction suppresses our immunity and increases our risk of getting an infection or cancer, or we could end up having a heart attack.

Yet at any time, we can choose to stop our hurt and suffering by learning to respond to potentially stressful situations in a positive way.

Anything we have learned we can unlearn. Whenever we experience emotional pain, it is because we have *learned* to respond to a certain situation in a negative way.

Yet we are completely free to choose a different response. Whenever we confront a life event, all we need to do is pause a moment before we react. Then instead of automatically replying with an angry distorted thought, this brief pause allows us to choose a calm, logical thought instead.

If fact, we can feel any way we want to feel at any time by choosing an appropriate thought and placing it in our mind. When someone says something that our belief system recognizes as insulting, we are perfectly free to respond with a cheerful and positive thought. Instead of automatically responding to a stimuli with an upsetting thought, we can respond with a thought that makes us feel good.

The best way to do it is to use stop-go switching (see Painstopper #96). In this case, though, you call out "Stop!" and you snap your rubber band whenever you must respond to a potentially stressful situation.

You need only call "Stop!" and snap your rubber band once. At this point, instead of automatically responding in a negative or hostile way, pause for a brief moment. Then choose a positive, cheerful, and love-based thought as your response.

When a person lashes out at you, what he or she really wants is recognition and love. So give them what they want. At the same time, you will be saving yourself from experiencing hurt, suffering, or emotional pain.

With a few exceptions, it's possible to enjoy every moment of every day and to feel positive and happy almost all the time.

"But I could never feel like that," one woman told me. "I need to have bad days in order to have something to compare my good days to. I'd just be a zombie if I felt positive all the time and never felt unhappy."

"Not so." I replied. "Most of us are zombies now. We have absolutely no freedom to choose our responses. When someone presses your emotional button A, tape X always begins to play. Press your emotional button B and tape Y will always start to play. Most of us are just like robots. Most of our responses are automatic, and we have absolutely no choice in the way we respond to external stimulus. Moreover, we'll go on being zombies until we take responsibility for our thoughts and feelings and learn that we *are* free to choose to feel any way we want to feel at any time."

To stop being an emotional zombie, identify the six life events you most commonly face, and to which you automatically respond in a negative way. Then write down a more appropriate, positive response to each one. Memorize these responses and use therapeutic imagery to rehearse your replies (see Painstopper #13).

Responding in the way we've been culturally conditioned may seem "natural." But all too often it's inappropriate and harmful to our health and well-being. When we choose to stop being an emotional zombie, and to liberate ourselves from our cultural conditioning, we can start to choose responses that make us feel good instead of responses that lead to emotional pain.

Cognitive Therapy Ends Emotional Pain in 7 Minutes Flat

Every Wednesday at the Women's Club Luncheon, Eleanor J. felt hurt and insulted by what she perceived as one woman's cutting remarks. For instance, Eleanor was proud of her new hair style until this woman remarked that it made her look much better. To Eleanor, this was a rude, sarcastic way of implying that previously, she must have looked worse.

This seemed like the last straw. Eleanor felt so hurt and depressed that she made an appointment with a psychotherapist.

The therapist recognized her problem as mild depression brought on by distorted thinking, and he prescribed cognitive therapy.

When Eleanor wore a new dress to the woman's club luncheon two weeks later, the same woman remarked, "This dress makes you look so much slimmer."

Eleanor immediately snapped her rubber band and silently called out, "Stop!" Instead of automatically feeling angry and hurt, Eleanor paused and deliberately chose her response.

Eleanor realized that she *could* have perceived the remark as implying that normally she appeared overweight. But Eleanor also recognized that it was not the woman's remark that was important but the way in which her own mind was handling it. This allowed her to graciously say, "Thank you, Dorothy, that's very nice."

By then, Eleanor was already beginning her five deep breaths. She implanted her seed thought-image, a beautiful garden scene in which she mentally experienced the calming scent of lilacs. Eleanor felt so calm, in fact, that she was able to recognize that her mind had been ignoring her many positive attributes and successes while it focused on this one woman's remarks. Her therapist had called it, "ignoring positive factors while you concentrate on negative points." Also, she recognized that she had allowed her mind to be run by the way she felt instead of by logical thinking.

For the first time, Eleanor also realized that Dorothy's remarks might *not* have been intentionally hurtful or sarcastic. When she got home, Eleanor used the zen temple technique (described in our Painstopper #21) to forgive Dorothy completely and unconditionally and to forgive herself as well for having judged Dorothy's remarks.

As she concluded this powerful mental imagery, Eleanor felt as though an enormous and oppressive burden had slipped from her shoulders. It took only 7 minutes for all traces of depression and emotional pain to vanish and to be replaced by feelings of cheerfulness and optimism. That was over three years ago. And Eleanor has not experienced a trace of emotional pain since.

Chapter 14

QUESTIONS AND ANSWERS ABOUT NATURAL PAIN RELIEF

The following questions and answers, recorded at lectures and workshops given by the author, may help you to understand and use behavioral medicine in relieving pain.

Q. Why haven't you mentioned do-it-yourself massage-type therapies such as acupressure, shiatsu, or reflexology for pain relief?

A. We do include acupressure in Painstoppers #37, #99, and #100. However, no really dependable studies have demonstrated that these therapies provide significant relief for any type of pain. And if and when they do relieve pain, it may be for a very limited time.

Moreover, the pressure points in the body are so numerous and complex that we simply don't have space in this book to illustrate their positions. Even then, it's easy to miss the exact location, in which case your efforts could be wasted.

Q. Could you briefly describe one example of how acupressure can relieve pain?

A. An acupressure action-step most people can use successfully is described in Painstopper #99.

PAINSTOPPER #99:
Stopping a Charleyhorse with Acupressure

A charleyhorse is a severe and painful spasm or cramping of the muscles in the upper or lower leg. It may last 2 or 3 minutes before disappearing. The cause is usually a deficiency of magnesium and other minerals in the diet.

Acupressure relief for a charleyhorse consists of seizing the mustache area between the thumb and finger of one hand and pinching it tightly until the cramped muscle releases. The mustache area of the face is the crease between the bottom of your nose and upper lip. Don't hurt yourself, but you must apply firm, steady pressure. Usually, this is enough to release the muscle spasm.

(In case this action-step fails, try to straighten your leg and pull the toes of your cramped leg back toward you. Of if you are standing, straighten the cramped leg and stand with the ball of your foot on a step so that the heel hangs down. Put your weight on this leg to lower the heel and pull out the spasm.)

Q. *You recommend that any pain be medically diagnosed before you try to relieve it. Suppose I must wait a week for a doctor's appointment. Is there any one technique I could use to relieve a pain of unknown origin?*

A. If you are able to exercise, a brisk walk of 35 minutes or more—brisk enough to raise your pulse and breathing rates significantly—is probably the one best all around pain reliever in existence (see Painstopper #2). Failing that, try the action-steps in Painstopper #100.

PAINSTOPPER #100:
To Relieve a Pain of Unknown Origin

The following action-steps are intended only to provide pain relief until your pain can be medically diagnosed. Steps 1, 2, and 3 should all be done simultaneously. Maintain them for up to 5 minutes at a time provided you can do so without discomfort. Stop any action-step immediately if it causes dizziness or discomfort. After resting for 20 minutes, you could repeat the three steps again. I suggest using them for a maximum of 10 minutes in each hour. Be careful not to become dizzy from deep breathing or to overdo the earlobe massage.

- *Step 1:* Gently but firmly hold your left earlobe between the thumb and forefinger of your left hand; hold your right earlobe between the thumb and forefinger of your right hand. Maintain *gentle* pressure as you use a circular motion to massage each earlobe between your thumb and forefinger. This action-step activates a number of acupressure points within each earlobe.

  You may want to maintain this earlobe massage for only a minute at a time. Rest a full minute before beginning again. Meanwhile, keep up steps 2 and 3 without pause.

- *Step 2:* Begin slow, deep belly breathing. As you inhale, fill the abdomen first and the upper chest last. Exhale in the opposite order. Abdominal breathing is explained in full in Painstopper #7. Slow, deep breathing relaxes the body and raises the pain threshold, thus diminishing the experience of any type of pain.

- *Step 3*: Ask yourself what shape your pain is. Close your eyes and visualize that shape in your mind's eye. Then, in your imagination, project that shape 10 feet out in front of you. Magnify the shape to ten times its original size. Next visualize it filled with water. You "see" a spigot at the bottom of the shape. Mentally, open the spigot and watch the water drain out.

  In your mind's eye, reduce the shape back to its original size. Then shrink it down to one-tenth that size. Return it to its original size. Fill the shape with a healing green light. Keeping it filled with the healing green light, magnify the shape to ten times its original size. Next, shrink it back down to one-tenth its original size—and still "see" it filled with healing green light. Then return it to its original size and move it back into your mind.

Painstopper #14 describes how to do this in greater detail and also explains that the brain activity you generate helps to close your neurological pain gate and to shut off pain impulses to your brain.

By functioning on the physical, psychological, and neurological levels simultaneously, these steps provide a holistic, or wide-spectrum, approach that is often more successful than working on one level of pain relief only.

Painstoppers #7 through #20 may also help to relieve a pain of unknown origin.

Q. *Is it possible to relieve chronic pain permanently without using a whole-person approach?*

A. Yes, some types of chronic pain can be permanently relieved by a single painstopper technique. But let's not forget that the underlying cause of most types of chronic pain is unresolved emotional stress that triggers the fight-or-flight response and sets off tension in the body muscles. This stress arises out of mental conflicts that occur when we hold inappropriate beliefs in our minds.

Many people who have suffered for years from lower back pain are able to clear it up and to prevent any further recurrence by practicing yoga-type stretches and by doing strength-building exercises on a daily basis. These people save their backs. But their stress and tension are still there. This tension might then begin to set off tension headaches. So instead of chronic back pain, a person may get chronic headaches. Whereas had he or she used a whole-person approach that included belief restructuring, that person could have been free of any kind of future pain.

Of course, using a whole-person approach, which typically includes three or four painstopper techniques, takes more time and effort than merely practicing a single technique. Yet the extra effort can be worthwhile. In addition to creating chronic pain, stress and tension can suppress immunity and increase a person's risk of getting cancer, heart disease, or a life-threatening infection like pneumonia.

So a few extra minutes a day spent reprogramming negative beliefs can pay off with greatly enhanced health and well-being.

Q. *What about natural ways for overcoming the pain of conditions such as prostate problems, TMJ headaches (a headache due to tension in the jaw or temporomandibular joint), cancer, pancreatitis, tumor of the spinal cord, or cluster headaches? I don't see these listed in this book.*

A. To begin, prostate problems, and some types of cancer, are often painless, while no really effective natural method may exist to relieve the pain of a cluster headache. Most TMJ headaches can be permanently relieved by having your dentist make a splint that you slip between your teeth at bedtime. Other conditions, such as pancreatitis or a tumor of the spine, may be so life threatening that using any type of physical action-step could be dangerous.

Nonetheless, mental action-steps, like relaxation training or therapeutic imagery, are highly effective against every type of mind-body pain, including cancer, pancreatitis, or a spinal tumor.

Q. If it is possible to avoid such painful diseases as angina or heart disease by using behavioral medicine, why are so many expensive heart bypass operations still being done each year?

A. A good question! Nowadays, the average bypass operation costs at least $40,000, and with medication, follow-ups, and rehabilitation, the bill often totals $100,000. There's still a significant risk of dying as a result of the operation. And a recent Rand Corporation study concluded that at least 30 percent of bypass operations were of debatable value, while another 14 percent were unjustified.

Moreover, unless behavioral medicine is also used—that means making major changes in diet and life-style—within five years half of all new bypass arteries may become blocked once more with fatty deposits. A fresh bypass operation every few years is commonplace. Reaming out blocked arteries with angioplasty or atherectomy operations is cheaper, but here again, up to 30 percent of arteries may become blocked again within six months.

By contrast, other studies show that up to 80 percent of all patients with angina pain or heart disease could recover completely by using behavioral medicine alone. That means changing our behavior. It means cutting out smoking and alcohol and replacing the typical high-fat, meat-based standard American diet with a low-fat, high-fiber diet of plant-based foods. It means following a healthful life-style that includes daily exercise and managing stress.

But as one woman told me, "Replacing steaks and ice cream with fruits and vegetables, or with peasant foods like millet or barley, or walking for exercise goes against our culture. Yet having a bypass or angioplasty operation, or going on cholesterol-lowering drugs for life, seems as American as apple pie."

"Besides," she added, "unless I have an operation, I have nothing to tell my friends about. They can understand something physical like blocked arteries. But what would they think if I told them I visualized myself in a Zen temple every day forgiving my enemies?"

As this was written, some 380,000 bypass operations were still being done in America each year. Assuming that 80 percent might have been avoided by using behavioral medicine, it means that every year, 304,000 people prefer to believe that they are helpless victims of heart disease pain instead of being willing to do what it takes to overcome their pain naturally.

Q. Isn't it easier to pop a pain pill than to do some of the painstopper techniques you suggest?

A. Yes, provided the pain pill doesn't produce any adverse side effects. The trouble is that every medication is a two-edged sword. One edge may help to relieve your pain. But if you begin to take the drug regularly, the other edge can produce such harsh side effects as vivid nightmares, hallucinations, vomiting and stomach upset, depression, bone loss, insomnia, or in some cases, even kidney failure, stroke, or heart disease. Even then, most OTC and prescription medications begin to lose their pain-killing potency after a week or two.

Relieving pain naturally by using your mind or muscles may take more time and effort. But side effects are zero, and the more you use them, the more effective these natural techniques become at killing pain.

Of course, some people should never even consider using the painstopper techniques in this book. And it's a safe bet that they will never try. Yet the average person can safely use behavioral medicine.

Q. If a person believes that a certain drug can relieve his pain, isn't the placebo effect responsible for at least some of this pain relief?

A. Yes. The placebo effect is the only natural pain-zapping power that can be released by a drug. Studies made to determine a drug's effectiveness take the placebo effect into consideration.

But if a drug is 90 percent effective in relieving a certain patient's pain, it still means that roughly one-third of that effect is due to the person's belief in the drug. In terms of chemical activity, the drug is only 60 percent effective in relieving that person's pain. The other 30 percent of pain relief emanates from the placebo effect.

Q. Can the painstopper action-steps in this book help a person suffering from the pain of terminal cancer?

A. Yes. Although some cancers are relatively pain-free, those that have spread to the bone — or in which a tumor exerts pressure on an adjacent nerve — can be excruciatingly painful.

Recent reports show that thousands of people with terminal cancer in American hospitals are given inadequate medication to relieve their pain.

The reason? The most powerful and successful painkilling drugs are narcotics. And many doctors hesitate to prescribe higher doses of narcotics because the state drug control bureau may regard them as promoting drug addiction. For similar reasons, in states that restrict controlled substances, millions of other hospital patients may also be given inadequate pain-relieving medication.

For anyone in this unfortunate situation, all the mental action-steps in this book—from Painstoppers #7 to #21—can be used to relieve the pain of terminal cancer, or of any other illness, disease, injury, or dysfunction.

Q. For applying heat or cold, isn't there something more modern than the old-fashioned icebag or a hot pack made by wrapping a loaf of bread inside a towel?

A. If you need to apply cold or moist heat for any length of time, it may pay to buy a modern hot wrap or cold wrap. These are gel packs with a 48-inch stretch fabric bandage and a Velcro® fastener. The cold wrap contains chemicals that deliver an instant freeze in just 30 seconds. It works only once. But afterward, you can store the cold wrap in the freezer and use it like a regular gel pack. Or pop the hot wrap in a microwave for a few minutes, and it will deliver two hours of moist heat. These hot and cold wraps are available in most drugstores and supermarkets.

Q. *Is it possible to tap into your subconscious mind for guidance about pain relief?*

A. This is a popular method at pain clinics nowadays. You will find it explained in Painstopper #101.

PAINSTOPPER #101:
Pain Relief Guidance from Within

For several months Hal J. had suffered from severe tension headaches and frequently occurring lower back pain. After failing to find anything wrong, his doctor referred Hal to a pain clinic. But the doctors there were also unable to come up with a diagnosis.

Finally, Hal was interviewed by the clinic's psychologist. The psychologist told Hal that he could probably find the answer he sought by contacting his "inner guide." Hal was to go into deep relaxation and then to visualize a small lawn covered by an opaque white cloud. As a puff of wind blew the cloud away, there, revealed on the lawn, would be Hal's "inner guide." The guide might be a person or an animal, for example, a wise old man or the earth mother, or a spiritual leader, a wise owl or crow, or a rabbit or other animal.

The psychologist explained that our "inner guide" is actually a symbol for our own deepest self. Our guide (meaning our inner self) has access to the deepest levels of our body-mind, including our memory banks.

Our guide can take us on a mental voyage of self-discovery into the depths of our subconscious or into the vast array of memories stored in our memory banks. A dialog with our inner guide can provide a penetrating insight about the source of any pain and about the best way to heal it.

The psychologist explained that the first thing Hal saw on the lawn when the cloud blew away would be his inner guide, and whenever he questioned his guide, the first thing that came into his mind would be the answer.

Hal's guide turned out to be a wise old man with a long white beard. After exchanging greetings, Hal learned that his guide's name was Methuselah. Hal asked Methuselah how his headaches and backaches were caused and how they could be relieved.

Methuselah replied by pointing to a rowboat tied up to the bank of a small lake. Hal and Methuselah got into the boat and Methuselah rowed out into the lake. Then Methuselah stood up and dived into the lake.

He remained submerged for nearly a minute. At last, his head broke the surface close to the boat. Methuselah reached up out of the water and handed a round white object to Hal.

"This is the cause of your pain," Methuselah said. Then he waved his hand and slid once more beneath the surface. This time, he did not reappear.

When Hal looked at the object Methuselah had given him, he saw that it was a large wall clock. But this clock had no hands. And the white face was completely blank.

Hal was puzzled. Could this be the answer to his pain? Suddenly, it came to him. His problem was hurry sickness. His fast-paced life-style was causing his headaches and back pain.

Hal realized that his life was run by the clock. He was always running late. Each day, his life was geared to meeting a series of schedules that even his Type A personality could never meet.

As Hal realized that Methuselah had indeed given him the guidance he sought, he experienced a mounting sense of relief. Starting next morning, Hal planned a more relaxed workday with fewer schedules and deadlines to meet. Hal was unable to learn whether his headaches and back pain had been due to tension or to a deeper cause. But he never experienced either type of pain again.

In subsequent visualization sessions, Hal was able to resume contact with Methuselah. And he has used Methuselah's advice to achieve a high level of fitness and health.

■ HOW TO MEET YOUR INNER GUIDE

Naturally, if you have any type of psychological problem, or if you are subject to schizophrenia or hallucinations or to any type of mental illness, you should not use this type of therapeutic imagery without the express permission of your doctor. Otherwise, here's how you can meet and consult with your own inner guide. (Before beginning, read Painstopper #13: Silence Pain with Therapeutic Imagery.)

- *Step 1:* Go into deep relaxation, using either Painstopper #9 or the speedier method in Painstopper #10.

- *Step 2:* Stay deeply relaxed and remain lying down with your eyes closed. Visualize a green lawn. The lawn is covered by an opaque white cloud about 9 feet high. A sudden gust of wind blows the cloud away. Your inner guide is revealed on the lawn.

- *Step 3:* Introduce yourself to your inner guide and ask the guide's name. One man's inner guide was a furry, white rabbit called Henry. As their inner guide, some people see themselves as a child.

- *Step 4:* Ask your guide how your pain is caused and what is causing it. The reply may come in words, intuition, a picture, or a symbol. You may be instructed to seek the answer in a certain book or magazine article. Or the answer may appear during a dream. Jot down details of the answer in a notebook. It may not make sense at first, but if you write it down, the answer may become apparent later. At the same time, note all your impressions and any shapes or colors that appear.

- *Step 5:* Ask your guide if it is possible to take your pain away, even if only for a few hours. Then ask what you yourself can do to relieve your pain.

- *Step 6:* Ask your guide what your pain is trying to tell you. Frequently, pain is a warning that you are overworking or overstressing yourself. Your guide may tell you to introduce more fun, pleasure, and enjoyment into your life. If your guide's advice makes sense and is obviously health enhancing, go ahead and use it if you can. If not, ask your guide if this is really what he, she, or it meant.

- *Step 7:* Thank your guide and ask for the swiftest way to re-establish contact. Or better yet, make an appointment to meet again at a certain hour and day. Ask that communication become faster, simpler, and easier. Then bid your guide goodbye.

■ A FINAL QUESTION

I'd like to conclude this book by answering the one question people most frequently ask me about pain:

Q. *Is it possible to go through life without ever experiencing any form of chronic pain?*

A. And my answer is a clear and resounding "Yes!"

Mind you, I'm talking about chronic, long-term pain not about acute pain from temporary causes like childbirth or a sprained ankle.

As we read a book like this, and learn more and more about chronic pain, few of us fail to be impressed by one obvious fact. At least 75 percent of all long-term pain is caused by the vicissitudes of our own life-style. We all know that four of every five smokers will die from the effects of smoking and that their deaths will be painful.

But until we learn the facts, few of us are aware that our flabby, unexercised muscles are responsible for millions of cases of lower back and knee pain. It's the standard American diet—high in fat and low in fiber—that keeps 40 percent of Americans overweight and that is responsible for other millions of cases of painful osteoarthritis, angina pain, and knee, hip, and back pain. Millions of other chronic pain cases can be traced to the extended use of over-the-counter or prescription drugs or to scar tissue from surgery that failed.

More incredible still is that millions of us keep on doing the very things that cause and perpetuate chronic pain. Making these risk factors difficult to avoid is that some have become an integral part of the American Dream while others are deeply ingrained in the American culture.

Nonetheless, if we're willing to make the effort we *can* make ourselves virtually painproof. All it takes is to drop, one by one, each of our pain-pro-voking habits and to replace each with a health-enhancing habit. With each step we take, we release pain-zapping powers that motivate us to break *all* our pain-reinforcing habits and to replace each of them with behaviors that lead to health and comfort.

To begin, we need only identify our most common and most dangerous pain-causing habits.

■ THE NINE LEADING CAUSES OF CHRONIC PAIN

1. Failing to engage in vigorous daily exertion that includes aerobic, strength-building, and stretching exercises.
2. Eating a high-fat, low-fiber diet high in dairy and flesh foods and refined carbohydrates instead of a low-fat, high-fiber diet of plant-based foods high in complex carbohydrates.
3. Indulging in smoking, chewing tobacco, recreational drugs, or more than two alcoholic drinks daily.
4. Engaging in the long-term use of OTC or prescription drugs and medications that are not really essential.
5. Failing to manage stress successfully.
6. Failing to provide the body with its biological requirements, such as adequate sleep, pure air and water, relaxation, quiet, emotional calm, sunshine, and security.
7. Overeating and obesity.
8. Holding fear-based beliefs that invoke such health-wrecking emotions as anger, envy, resentment, anxiety, depression, or frustration.
9. Believing you are a passive, helpless victim of pain and disease and being unwilling to do what it takes to maintain optimal health at all times.

■ WE CAN CHOOSE TO BE PAIN-FREE

Endless case histories and studies show that when a person eliminates from his or her life-style the nine causes of chronic pain just listed, chances are good that chronic pain will never occur. There's also a better than even chance that by eliminating these destructive habits, any chronic pain you already have may also gradually disappear.

To remain pain-free for life, we merely need to adopt the health-restoring advice already spelled out in such Painstoppers as #2: Walk Away from Pain, #3: The One Diet that Does it All, #9: Relaxation Training, and #21: Keep Pain at Bay with Positive Beliefs.

So there's really nothing holding us back. Each of us is entirely free to choose to use our minds and muscles to create a life-style that is completely incompatible with the existence of chronic pain.

Index

A

Abdominal breathing, 29, 60-62, 71-73, 89, 105, 178, 271
Action-steps, 8-9
    classes of, 39-40
Action therapy. *See* Behavioral medicine
Active therapy, 6-7, 79, 132
Acupressure, 169, 269-271
Age, 41
Albany Medical College, 145
American Psychology Association, 78
Angina, 19, 46, 48, 50, 214-218, 273, 279
Annals of Internal Medicine, 132
Arthritis, 8, 45, 127-149
    osteo-, 27, 55, 110, 134-243
    rheumatoid, 25, 45-46, 93, 99, 121, 128-137, 143-149
Arthritis Foundation, 45

B

Beck, Aaron T., 259
Behavioral medicine, 2-3, 7, 11, 26, 31, 116, 129, 167, 195, 216, 258, 273-274
Belief restructuring, 26-27, 39, 115-125
Belief system, 25-26, 32-33
Benson, Dr. Herbert, 28
Bicycling, benefits of, 45-46
    for arthritis, 133
    for headaches, 167-169
Biofeedback, 11, 29, 39, 73-78, 100, 178-179, 258
Bland, John H., 132
Bodymind connection, 12, 13, 32, 35-36, 40, 61, 256
    See also Whole person approach
Boston University School of Medicine and Medical Center, 141, 144
Brainwaves, 61-63
Brigham and Women's Hospital, Boston, 145

Bristol Myers and Company, 41
British Medical Journal, 186, 248
Burns, David D., 259
Bursitis, 153-157

C

Calcium, 28, 218
Cancer, 25, 48, 185, 209, 272, 275
Case Western Reserve, 181
Charleyhorse, relieving, 270
Chicago Medical School, 58
Cognitive therapy, 259-267
Chronic benign pain syndrome, 1, 35
    phantom pain, 35
City of London Migraine Clinic, 186
Claudication, 214-216, 219
Creative imagery. *See* Therapeutic imagery

D

Depression, 26, 30, 256-267, 274
Diamond Headache Clinic, Chicago, 75, 169
Diary keeping, 51-55
Diffusing pain, 111
Distorted thinking, 259-267
Distorting time, 113-114
Diverticulosis, 56-57, 210-211
Drugs, painkilling, 3, 279
    side effects of, 3-4, 274

E

Eastern Tennessee State University, 181
Emotional pain, 255-267
Emotions, negative, 32-33, 35, 115, 121-122, 148-149, 155-267
Emotions, positive, 25-26, 116, 122-125
Enabling effect, 15, 31, 54-55, 79
Endorphins, 16, 34-35, 44-45, 47, 79, 104-106

Lifestyle habits that relieve pain, 18, 43, 151-
152, 279
Li-shou technique, 161-164
Lorig, Dr. Kate, 8
Lower back pain, 12, 25-26, 45, 189-208, 214,
272, 276-279
Lupus, 129

M

Magnesium, 19-20, 50, 180-183, 218
Massage, 173-176
for lower back pain, 192
for sinusitis, 244
for tic douleureux, 242
Mayo Clinic, 73, 219
McGill University, Canada, 169
McKnight, Peggy, 146
Medically-informed layperson, 8-9, 138, 215-216
Melzack, Robert, 169
Menninger Institute, Topeka, Kansas, 64, 73
Mental imagery. *See* Therapeutic imagery
Mind as pain reliever, 10-11, 36, 75, 82
Music to soothe pain, 78

N

National Center for Health Statistics, 165
National Institute for Clinical Application of Be-
havioral Medicine, 116
Natural pain-relieving mechanisms (pain-zap-
ping powers), 5-7, 11, 14, 20-21, 23, 79
Neck pain, 232-237
Nerve fibers, 30-31, 240
Neural pain, 237-242
Neuropeptides, 32
Norepinephrine (noradrenalin), 28-29, 31, 34

O

Ornish, Dean, 216

P

Pain clinics, 12
Pain color, 83, 86, 91-92, 96-98

Pain gate, 15, 29-31, 79, 101-104, 170-171, 271
Pain mechanism, 24-37
Pain object, 83, 86, 91-92, 96, 98
Pain relief color, 83, 88, 91-92, 98
Pain relief imagery. *See* Therapeutic imagery
Pain relief object, 83, 88, 91-92, 98
Painstopper, defined, 39-41
Passive therapy, 6
Perception of pain, changing your, 108-109
Phenylalanine, 30
Physiatrist, 5, 194
Placebo effect, 9, 14-15, 24, 36-37, 79, 274-275
Pritikin Program, 217
Projecting pain away, 112-113
Prostaglandin, 28-29, 152
Purines, 149-152

R

Rand Corporation, 273
Relaxation training, 11, 29, 34, 39, 59-73, 75,
77, 89, 100, 258, 273
aids and audiotapes for, 77
Reticular system neural pathway, 34-35
Right brain language, 10, 34, 86, 95
Royal Adelaide Hospital, Australia, 146
Royal Victoria Hospital, Montreal, 78

S

St. Margaret's Memorial Hospital, Pittsburgh, 146
Sargent, Joseph, 64
Sciatica, 248-254
Selback, Patricia, 64
Serotonin, 30-31, 34, 47-48, 50
Shoes, ill-fitting, 225
Shoulder pain, 232-237
Sinusitis pain, 242-244
Stanford University, 8
Stop-Go Switching, 55-58, 141, 262-263, 265
Straight line neural pathway, 33
Stress, 24-26, 29, 41, 148, 193, 218, 255-257,
272, 280
Stretching exercise. *See also* Yoga